GLOSSARY of
GROUP and
FAMILY
THERAPY

GLOSSARY of GROUP and FAMILY THERAPY

Edward L. Pinney, Jr., M.D.

and

Samuel Slipp, M.D.

BRUNNER/MAZEL • New York

Library of Congress Cataloging in Publication Data

Pinney, Edward Lowell, 1925-
  Glossary of group and family therapy.

  1. Group psychotherapy—Terminology.
2. Family psychotherapy—Terminology.
I. Slipp, Samuel. II. Title. [DNLM:
1. Psychotherapy, Group—Dictionaries.
2. Family therapy—Dictionaries. WM 13 P656g]
RC488.P56   616.89′15′0321   82-4193
ISBN 0-87630-300-9   AACR2

Copyright © 1982 by Edward L. Pinney, Jr., and Samuel Slipp

Published by
BRUNNER/MAZEL, INC.
19 Union Square West
New York, New York 10003

MANUFACTURED IN THE UNITED STATES OF AMERICA

To my teachers at the schools, universities and hospitals where I have studied. They prepared me to learn from my patients.

E.L.P.

To my wife Sandra and my daughter Elena, whose love and encouragement enabled this book to be possible, and to my dear friends who have remained in my memory as a living inspiration, Peter Hogan, Don Jackson, Alfred Rifkin, Jack Royce, Albert Scheflen, and Sheldon Selesnick

S.S.

Editorial Advisory Board

Contents

Introduction

We could not write a Glossary without reference to "the great lexicographer," Samuel Johnson, who published his monumental dictionary of the English language in 1755. Indeed, our six research assistants busying themselves collecting and diligently writing down items called to mind the image of the six assistants Johnson employed in his attic in London. With Johnson as our guide, we were comforted, especially during difficult and perplexing times, by his comment, "Dictionaries are like watches: the worst is better than none, and the best cannot be expected to go quite true." We realized we could attempt but could not achieve perfection. We were spurred on by the need for clear working definitions of terms, as well as biographical sketches of pioneers and leaders, in the fields of group and family therapy.

Since World War II, group therapy has expanded from a form of therapy primarily used because of lack of trained professionals and for economic reasons to an important form of psychotherapy that can stand firmly on its own merits. Family therapy, which is only slightly over 20 years old, has also grown enormously and mushroomed into a broad and popular field employing various therapeutic approaches. We have limited this Glossary to terms that are used specifically in group and family therapy. Because of the continued growth in these two psychotherapeutic approaches, new knowledge, new techniques, and thus new terms have been constantly evolving. The language of group and family therapy is a living language. New terms are born and old terms may disappear or acquire new meanings. Thus, no glossary can ever be complete as long as the field is dynamic and alive.

Making decisions about including terms, organizations, journals, and individuals contributing to these two fields of group and family therapy was no easy task. We were aware we might be criticized by some and we recognized that others would disagree with the judgments we made to include or exclude certain items. Each member of the Editorial Advisory Board received a copy of the draft of the Glossary and was also consulted individually on specific areas in order to validate our judgments. Our hope was thus to minimize or eliminate any personal bias that may have been introduced outside of our conscious awareness. While we have every reason to believe that our definitions and other inclusions in the Glossary will generally be accepted by our professional colleagues, we do welcome suggestions for revisions or additions for future editions of the Glossary.

Samuel Johnson defined a rambler as a pompous, affected writer who never used a short English word if he could find a long Latin one to put in its place. Thus brevity was held by us as a virtue and a guide. There were three other qualities we sought after in making this dictionary: accuracy, clarity, and comprehensiveness. No definitions were simply taken from any other glossary. Each term was researched by us and our research assistants from original sources in journals and books. If errors were to be made, at least they were to be our own. We attempted to glean the most frequently used terms that occur in the literature for group and family therapy. We felt that significant people currently working in the fields of group and family therapy and those who contributed in the past should be included. Taking the entries to our Editorial Advisory Board and considering their suggestions led to our final draft.

This process resulted in what we believe is the first comprehensive glossary in the areas of group and family therapy. Our aim was to standardize the meaning and usage of terms which we felt would satisfy the needs of those in the field. We hope it will facilitate greater dialogue and development in group and family therapy, prevent misunderstandings, and be of practical use to therapists.

Most of all, our thanks go to all members of our Editorial Advisory Board, who gave generously of their time and were constructive in their comments and recommendations.

Edward L. Pinney, Jr.
Samuel Slipp

Acknowledgments

Our special thanks go to the Spanish-speaking members of our Editorial Advisory Board who have gone to some trouble to call our attention to glossaries for group psychotherapy in other languages. In this regard Dr. A. G. Gomez, Dr. Juan Rossello, and, through Dr. Gomez, Dr. Edmundo Ruiz have been most generous. Dr. Lyman Wynne made generous contributions to the family therapy section.

We wish to thank the New York University fieldwork placement research assistants, as well as Madeline Cylkowsky, Lewis Levy, Hope Aspell, and Diane Pinney.

GLOSSARY of GROUP and FAMILY THERAPY

Group
Therapy
Section

Abell, Richard G.
   American psychiatrist and psychoanalyst, who is on the faculty of William A. White Institute. He wrote the ABC-TV national network series "Road to Reality" based on group psychotherapy sessions. He founded the Transactional Analysis Institute of New York and Connecticut and is the author, with Corliss W. Abell, of *Own Your Own Life*, Bantam, New York, 1977.

Ackerman, Nathan W. (1908-1971) (See Family Therapy Section)
   American psychiatrist and psychoanalyst. An early innovator in group and pioneer of family psychotherapy. Training analyst at Columbia Psychoanalytic Institute. Founder and Director of the Ackerman Institute for Family Therapy in New York City. Author of the first textbook of family therapy, *The Psychodynamics of Family Life*, Basic Books, New York, 1958, and with Don Jackson originated the first family therapy journal, *Family Process*.

action group (A-group)
   A group whose task is to discuss and solve a problem and develop a program for action. It is common in community and business organizations.

activity group therapy

A type of group therapy designed primarily for children and adolescents, which by use of group activities, games, and dancing affords an outlet for repressed emotions. S. R. Slavson and Mortimer Schiffer are leading exponents of activity group therapy.

adapted child

A term used in transactional analysis to indicate the child ego state which functions submissively to parental influences as opposed to the free or natural child.

Adler, Alfred (1870-1937)

Viennese psychiatrist and psychoanalyst, an early associate of Freud. He developed the concepts of inferiority complex and overcompensation.

Adler used group techniques in 1918 when he organized and conducted child guidance clinics for problem children in the public school system of Vienna.

affection phase

In the last stage of an ideal psychotherapy group, the members of the group feel affection towards the therapist and towards one another and express their feelings, both positive and negative, freely and spontaneously. In this stage, dependency and aggressive feelings are minimal.

affective honesty

A term devised by Hugh Mullan to denote an immediate emotional response to an authentic communication which admits that one has been reached.

affectualizing

A term that refers to going through the motions of expressing a feeling rather than actually experiencing a genuine feeling or emotion.

alternate meeting or alternate session (See coordinated
    meeting)
    A planned or regularly scheduled meeting of a psychotherapy
group without a therapist. This meeting is held alternately with
the meeting led by the therapist. Alternate meetings were originated by Alexander Wolf and made a part of his group treatment. There is no fee charged.

American Group Psychotherapy Association
    A professional multidisciplinary organization of over 3,000
members consisting of clinically qualified psychiatrists, psychologists, social workers, psychiatric nurses, and other mental
health professionals experienced in group psychotherapy—or
people who are unusually gifted and have made distinct contributions to group therapy and research. The organization was
originated in 1943 by Nathan W. Ackerman, Saul Bernstein,
Elizabeth Hobbie (representing Dr. Lowrey), George Holland,
G. Pederson-Krag, Harris B. Peck and S. R. Slavson. The Association has grown to become the organizational representative
of current group psychotherapy theory and practice in the
United States. The goals of the association are to encourage the
development of sound training programs in group psychotherapy, to establish and maintain high ethical and professional
standards in its practice, and to encourage research in the field.

analytic group psychotherapy
    Group psychotherapy for adults in which the therapist's in-
terventions follow psychoanalytic principles and techniques.
Psychoanalytic concepts of resistance, transference, and free
association are used, as well as dream interpretation. The goals
are developing insight, understanding unconscious origins of
current behavior, and working through to achieve behavioral
change.

antirepression device
    A technique used in encounter groups to gain access quickly

and directly to patients' feelings. Antirepression devices are usually nonverbal and involve physical contact. Some encounter "games" fall into this category.

Aronson, Marvin L.

American psychologist and psychoanalyst who has been the Director of Group Therapy at Postgraduate Center for Mental Health, New York, from 1971 to the present. He is the author of many papers in group therapy, especially on combined and conjoint treatment, and the book, *How to Overcome Your Fear of Flying*, Hawthorn Books, New York, 1971. In addition, from 1974-1979 he was the editor (with Lewis R. Wolberg) of the yearly book, *Group Therapy: An Overview*, published by Grune and Stratton, and since 1980 he has co-edited (also with Lewis R. Wolberg) the annual series, *Group and Family Therapy*, published by Brunner/Mazel.

art therapy in groups

A type of group treatment that uses painting and drawing by the group members as the essential part of the group work.

assembly phase

Ross Speck's term in network therapy for the meeting where all of the large group of friends, relatives, helpers or neighbors of the patient first assemble in a large group session.

assertiveness training group (see consciousness-raising group)

A group that helps members develop their ability to be assertive effectively. Techniques of assertiveness are taught didactically and members are shown how to maintain their rights in dealing with everyday interpersonal relationships. Behavioral therapy principles are usually followed in an assertiveness training group.

"assistant therapist" ("doctor's assistant," "helpful hannah," "therapist surrogate")

The role assumed by a group member who acts on his or her

own volition as assistant to the therapist to make interpretations, to question members of the group, and to take over the functions of the leader as he or she sees them.

Playing this role may be due to conscious altruism and a desire to help or to unconscious hostility and rivalry with the therapist. Denial of dependency needs and other inappropriate feelings sometimes motivate a patient to take up this role.

attraction (to the group)

A term that refers to the cohesion or pulling together of a group as indicated by the frequency of intra-group contacts and the intimacy of relationships, both emotional and intellectual.

attractiveness of the group (See cohesion)

Attractiveness refers to the value of the goals of the group when the group satisfies the needs of its members. It refers also to the individual attraction that the members feel for one another.

In *Group Dynamics: Research and Theory*, 2nd Ed., Harper & Row, New York, 1960, Cartwright and Zander listed the following factors that make a group attractive to its members:

1) Members are valued and accepted.
2) Members are similar.
3) The group is small enough so that members can communicate and relate effectively.
4) The group provides opportunities for social life and close personal associations.
5) At least two of the three following satisfactions are provided: personal attraction, task attraction, and prestige from membership.

auxiliary ego (See psychodrama)

In psychodrama, a therapist or assistant therapist functions as the patient's auxiliary ego when he or she takes the role of an important figure in the patient's life or a symbolic mental process, and voices a delusion or hallucination, the patient's unconscious wishes, guilt feelings, or unacceptable aspects of the self. The aim is to help the patient hear and understand his dissociated feelings and thinking.

Bach, George R.
American psychologist who developed a concept of group psychotherapy based on Kurt Lewin's field theory. Bach felt that the doctor must be group-oriented rather than only patient-oriented; he treats the patient by conscientiously creating an atmosphere that stimulates self-treatment. He is the author of many papers and the book, *Intensive Group Psychotherapy*, Ronald, New York, 1954.

basic assumption activity (See contagion; pairing)
In his work with group psychotherapy, Wilfred Bion observed that every group takes on or assumes automatic, unconscious reactions which he called basic assumption activities. These occur unconsciously, concurrently, and interfere with the task or goals that the group is working on. Basic assumption activities are readily seen in a group with a passive therapist, as structural organization diminishes and ambiguity emerges with respect to role definition. In their frustration, the group reacts against the therapist. Bion classifies a basic assumption activity as demonstrating flight or fight, pairing, or dependency activity (see Bion, Wilfred: *Experiences in Groups*. New York: Basic Books, 1960). It corresponds to the interference with higher ego functioning by regression to lower level impulses and needs.

basic skills training
A part of the training sessions in human relations which emphasizes leadership functions, communications skills, and the use of group process. National Training Laboratories was a leader in developing concepts of experiential learning, i.e., learning skills by doing instead of hearing about them.

Battegay, Raymond
Swiss psychiatrist well-known in international group psy-

chotherapy. Dr. Battegay is Chief of the Basle University Psychiatric Outpatient Clinic; Professor and Chairman (ad personam) of Psychiatry, Basle University; Past President, Swiss Medical Society for Psychotherapy; Past President, Commission for Social Psychiatry of the Swiss Psychiatric Association; Fellow of the American Academy of Psychoanalysis; Immediate Past President, International Association of Group Psychotherapy; and Board Member, International Association of Social Psychiatry.

Dr. Battegay is the author of several books including *Der Mensch in der Gruppe* (The Human Being in the Group), Vol. I, 1967/1976, Vol. II, 1967/1973, Vol. III, 1969/1979; *Der Mensch in der Gruppe* (The Human Being in the Group) shortened version as pocket-book, 1974; *Gruppenpsychotherapie und klinische Psychiatrie* (Group Psychotherapy and Clinical Psychiatry), 1963. Corresponding Editor, *International Journal of Group Psychotherapy* and author of 390 scientific publications on group psychotherapy, theory of neuroses and medical psychology, borderline situations, aggression, narcissism, anxiety, psychopathology, psychopharmacology, alcohol, and drug-dependencies.

Beckenstein, Nathan
American psychiatrist. President, American Group Psychotherapy Association, 1958-1960.

behavioral group therapy
In this type of group therapy the members pay more attention to overt observable behavior, especially symptomatic behavior, than to repressed thoughts and feelings. The aim of this treatment is to change the behavior that causes suffering and maladjustment. Conditioning and teaching techniques are used predominantly. Attention is focused on one individual at a time rather than on the group process.

behind-the-back technique
A technique used in encounter groups in which one member sits with his/her back to the group and describes himself or herself to the group. Other members of the group then discuss

this person as if he or she were not present. Subsequently, the member turns around and participates in the group discussion.

Bennis, Warren
American psychologist, consultant on business administration, and educational administrator. He wrote many of the original articles on T-Groups, change theory, organizational practice, and was prominent in National Training Laboratories. The author of books on many topics, including organizational structure and group process.

Berger, Irving L.
American psychiatrist. President, American Group Psychotherapy Association, 1978-1980.

Berger, Milton M.
American psychiatrist and psychoanalyst. President, American Group Psychotherapy Association, 1962-1964. Co-author with Max Rosenbaum of *Group Psychotherapy and Group Function*, ʹ Basic Books, New York, 1975, and *Beyond the Double Bind*, Brunner/Mazel, New York, 1980.

Berne, Eric (1910-1970)
American psychiatrist and founder of transactional analysis. He formulated the concept that our personality is composed of three ego states: Parent, Adult, and Child. From this he developed the concepts of life "script," early decision and redecision, injunctions, counter injunctions, reparenting, transactions, contracts, "strokes" and "games." He applied these concepts to the understanding of emotional conflicts and the treatment of psychopathology. Author of *Transactional Analysis in Psychotherapy*, Grove Press, New York, 1961, *Games People Play*, Grove Press, New York, 1964, and *Principles of Group Treatment*, Oxford University Press, New York, 1966.

Bierer, Joshua
Adlerian-trained English psychiatrist, who introduced the

practice of day-night hospitals and social clubs. Founder, International Association of Social Psychiatry. Editor, *International Journal of Social Psychiatry*.

bioenergetic group psychotherapy

Alexander Lowen's term for a type of group activity that uses physical exercises and nonverbal expressions of feelings to mobilize bodily energy. It is predicated on the theory that psychological symptoms result from bound-up muscle tension.

Bion, W. R. (1896-1980) (See basic assumption activity)

English psychiatrist and psychoanalyst. Author of *Experiences in Groups*, Basic Books, New York, 1961. Kleinian psychoanalytic theoretician known for his theories about therapy groups, i.e., Tavistock Groups, and who strongly influenced group therapy in South America.

Bion's innovative work was in group process and object relations theory, contributing the concept of "the container" for projective identification. He also pioneered the use of open wards in mental hospitals and the therapeutic milieu.

Blay-Neto, Bernardo

Brazilian psychiatrist who has made several contributions to the literature on countertransference and group work with special populations. He is a past president of the Federacao Latino Americana de Psicoterapia Analitica de Grupo.

blind walk

An encounter group technique that encourages feelings of trust within the group. Each member of the group chooses a partner and leads him or her around with the partner's eyes closed. The pair then exchange the roles of blind man and leader, and finally all reassemble as a group to discuss their reactions.

body contact maneuver (See encounter group therapy; activity group therapy)

Any technique that involves touching. Members of the group

touch or hold one another and then speak about the feelings aroused.

body language (See nonverbal communication;
        irrelevant action)
The way that a person's physical appearance, mannerisms, and gestures, as well as facial expressions, express a person's feelings and thinking. This is also called the science of kinesics.

boundary
A general systems theory term meaning the location where one system or sphere of activity ends and another begins. For instance, the school system for a first grader includes all that directly pertains to the activities of school for the pupil (i.e., the school itself, other pupils, homework, etc.). Where that system and another impinge (for instance, in homework where the home system and school system come together) would be the boundary of both systems. Boundary implies contact as such, or separating one set of activities and another.

breakthrough phase
Ross Speck's term for the phase in network therapy in which members see workable solutions to problems and ways that their efforts can be effective.

bull session
A leaderless informal group meeting in a social setting, such as a group of college students talking about an upcoming test. While not ostensibly therapeutic, bull sessions have anxiety-relieving and insight-producing effects.

Burling, Temple
American psychiatrist. President, American Group Psychotherapy Association, 1946-1947.

Burrow, Trigant (1875-1951)
American psychiatrist and psychoanalyst who did "phylo-

analysis" with groups. Burrow was a pioneer in utilizing group methods for treatment of personality problems which he felt were the product of current social forces. Author of *Science and Man's Behavior*, Philosophical Library, New York, 1953. A Summary Note on the Work of Trigant Burrow by Hans Syz (*International Journal of Social Psychiatry*, 1960, pp. 283-91) describes his work.

call system (See going-around)
Calling on each patient in turn at a group session to discuss specific issues.

captive group (See open group; free group)
A term used by Edward Pinney referring to a group that is confined to an institution or where attendance at group sessions is compulsory.

Carmichael, Donald M.
American psychiatrist. President, American Group Psychotherapy Association, 1954-1956.

catalytic agent
A term taken from chemistry and used by S. R. Slavson for those members of a group who stimulate the reactions of other members of the group but do not take part in the reactions or express their own feelings.

Christ, Jakob
Swiss psychiatrist who came to the United States in 1952 and was active in developing and directing group psychotherapy programs. Officer, American Group Psychotherapy Association and local group psychotherapy organizations. Moved to Switzerland from U.S. in 1979, where he developed local community mental health services.

class method
The Boston internist, Joseph Henry Pratt, called his method

of didactic group treatment the "class method." He modeled it on the Methodist Sunday School classes in Bible study and preferred this term to "group psychotherapy." In the early part of this century Dr. Pratt used the class method in the treatment of mental and physical illnesses.

client-centered therapy

A term defined by Carl Rogers in his book, *Client-Centered Counseling and Therapy*, Riverside Press, Cambridge, Mass., 1941. In this therapy, emphasis centers on the empathic discussion and understanding of material presented by client rather than the therapist's interventions.

closed group

A psychotherapy group in which the number of members remains unchanged throughout the series of sessions. No new members are added to the group, and the members selected at the beginning of the sessions are expected to remain with the group for a definite period of time or definite number of sessions.

cohesion (See attractiveness of the group)

Ronald D. Fairbairn used the term in 1935 to apply to the erotically oriented sociopsychological pressures that cause a group to stay together. Yalom in 1970 defined cohesion as the attraction of a group for its members, again citing erotic factors as opposed to hostile or destructive trends. Social psychologists give more importance to a common goal or a common danger as motivating cohesion in a group.

combined therapy (See conjoint therapy)

Treatment which uses both group and individual psychotherapy concurrently with the *same* therapist.

complementarity of interaction

Input of a group member that provokes an opposite or related reaction in response from other members. The reactions are highly specific to the character pathology and defensive structures of both the inducer of the interaction and the induced. For example, a masochistic patient may provoke an attacking response.

composition of a group (See group composition; group balance)
A term that refers to the kinds of patients selected for a group. A homogeneous group is made up of members who have qualities in common. A heterogeneous group contains a mixture of different types of patients.

The number of patients in a group should be neither too few nor too many. Four is considered the minimum number and the maximum usually 12. S. R. Slavson felt that eight was the maximum number of patients for a therapy group.

A group requires a degree of similarity in socioeconomic, ethnic and language background and a degree of similarity in psychopathology. The group may be composed entirely of psychotic patients, or a neurotic group may have one or at most two psychotics.

Selection of patients who "mirror" one another in behavior is considered helpful in group composition. When a compulsive, controlling mother is a patient, it is useful to have another compulsive, controlling mother in the group as her "mirror."

concretization of living (See psychodrama)
A technique that uses psychodrama to act out actual life experiences.

conductor (See social network therapy)
In social network therapy, the conductor is the team leader who helps catalyze the work of the network or tribe assembly. S. H. Foulkes used the term "conductor" to refer to the therapist of a therapeutic group.

congruence within a group (See body language)
The matching of verbal expression and actual feelings in a

group. Group members become aware of the discrepancies be-tween body language and verbal language in the process of developing congruence in a group.

conjoint therapy (See combined therapy)
Therapy in which the patient is in group and individual psy-chotherapy with different therapists for each type of treatment.

consciousness-raising group
A group designed to make a special selected group of people consciously aware of certain aspects relating to their social roles and their attitudes about them. This group is usually led by a nonprofessional, though members may meet without a leader. An example would be a group of women meeting to discuss how social conditions have affected them personally. A con-sciousness-raising group is not a psychotherapy group but can function as a support group for its members.

consensual observation
Trigant Burrow's term for consensual validation.

consensual validation (See universalization)
A term originated by Harry Stack Sullivan. Patients compare their reactions to certain life experiences with the reactions of others and learn that their emotional problems and mental op-erations are not unique and that they share the same experiences and problems with other people. When they compare their thoughts and feelings with the thoughts and feelings of others, they feel more certain about themselves. Their own reactions are supported by these comparisons, and self-confidence is en-hanced by this experience of reality-testing.

contagion (See basic assumption activity)
A group phenomenon in which the entire group becomes affected by a primitive emotional reaction. For example, anxiety can spread throughout a group and may widen to a level of panic. This occurs when the functioning of the group has been

pushed to a regressed level by either external or internal factors, and individuals are more suggestible or open. The term may be limited to mutual influences of affect or in a broader sense relate to unconscious conflicts. Individually, a group member may have a fear of contagion of mental illness, or an anxiety feeling about joining a group, or a fear of becoming sicker.

contamination
A term from transactional analysis that refers to the situation in which an aspect of the Child or Parent ego state—prejudice, assumption or habit of thinking—is accepted as fact by the Adult ego state, when actually it does not represent present reality.

contract
An agreement between patients and therapist that sets out the obligations and expectations of all concerned in a treatment situation. In group psychotherapy, resistance is expressed by failure to live up to the contract. Elements commonly considered essential to a contract for group psychotherapy are policies on meeting place, punctuality, addition of members, discharge of members, attendance, fees, outside group contracts of members, confidentiality, and manner of participation in the group.

coordinated meeting (See alternate meeting)
The term refers to a meeting without a therapist. It is also called an alternate meeting, a post-meeting session, and a pre-meeting session. Some therapists plan these meetings as an integral part of the therapy.

Coriat, Isador H. (1875-1943)
American psychiatrist and psychoanalyst who worked with Worcester and McComb at the Emmanuel Church in Boston on their "Health Conference," the first group psychotherapy meeting for nervous and mental disorders in 1906. Co-author with Worcester and McComb of *Religion and Medicine*, Moffat-Yard, New York, 1908.

Corsini, Raymond J.

American psychologist affiliated with the Industrial Relations Center, University of Chicago and the Chicago Community Child Guidance Center. Author of *Methods of Group Psychotherapy*, McGraw-Hill, New York, 1957.

counseling group (See task-oriented group)

Group that is limited to current reality issues and focuses on problem-solving. A counseling group has a specific purpose or a specific topic to discuss. Although a counseling group has some elements of a therapy group it is task-oriented and is usually limited to less than 10 sessions. The focus is on conscious concerns in contrast to unconscious conflicts or group process.

countertransference in group psychotherapy

A term referring to the unconscious projections of the therapist towards the members of his therapy group. These projections may stem from the therapist's own unsolved unconscious conflicts, or they may be stimulated by the behavior of any of the members of the group via projective identification, or by the behavior of the group as a whole.

couples group therapy

Group psychotherapy in which the group is composed of married couples or otherwise committed couples.

crisis intervention group therapy (See life transition group)

Group psychotherapy in which the participants work to ameliorate the effects of a specific recent emotional upheaval with which they have had difficulty coping. A crisis intervention group in group psychotherapy is usually limited to a few sessions but it may lead to long-term treatment.

crystalization

A term from transactional analysis that refers to a complementary transaction, Adult to Adult, between therapist and patient. It originates in the Adult ego state of the therapist and is received by the Adult ego state of the patient.

Curran, Frank J.
American psychiatrist who pioneered group psychotherapy for adolescents with Paul Schilder and Loretta Bender at Bellevue Hospital. In 1938 Frank Curran, along with Paul Schilder, S. R. Slavson and C. P. Oberndorf, belonged to the first group psychotherapy society.

dance therapy (See activity group therapy)
The use of dance and related body movement in treatment.

decision (See script)
A term from transactional analysis that refers to a firm commitment in early childhood to a specific life-style that persists into adult life. Early in life, children develop a plan for adaptation and survival. The plan is based on the way they are treated by their parents and the injunctions they receive from them. It determines whether they will be outgoing or withdrawn, happy or sad, winners or losers.

decontamination
In transactional analysis, decontamination refers to the removal of irrational Parent and Child ego state material from the Adult ego state of patients.

deflection
In a psychotherapy group one member shifts attention away from him- or herself to another member of the group. Deflection is a form of resistance.

deviance from group norm
Variation from accepted behavior or attitude in a group is termed deviance. Malcolm Pines defines deviance as lack of development of trust, lack of self-revelation, or continuing unre-

sponsiveness in a group member as the group progresses.

A group member who differs from other group members in socioeconomic status, ethnic or language background, or in psychopathology may also be called a deviant from the group norm.

didactic group psychotherapy

Group psychotherapy in which the intervention of the leader is actively educational and tutorial. The therapist brings up topics for discussion and outlines principles of mental hygiene and general principles of healthful living. J. M. Klapman is associated with this method. The aim of this method is intellectual understanding of mental and social problems.

direct soliloquy

A psychodrama technique in which a participant, while playing a role in the drama, steps aside and speaks his thoughts and feelings in a self-presentation to the group.

directive-didactic group psychotherapy

The first type of group psychotherapy used with institutional patients. Directive-didactic group therapy includes lectures by the therapist, group singing, and other activities suggested by the therapist. L. Cody Marsh was an early practitioner of this form of group psychotherapy.

In another type of directive-didactic group psychotherapy, the patients present problems and autobiographic material for the therapist and other patients to discuss.

directive-didactic psychodrama

A group treatment in which patients act out autobiographic material or material that is supplied by the therapist. Regressed patients in institutions are apt to benefit from this approach.

directive group psychotherapy

In directive group psychotherapy an active didactic leader takes charge and leads the activities and discussions of the group.

"doctor's assistant" (See "assistant therapist")

dominant member (See "assistant therapist," "helpful hannah")

The member of a group who tends to dominate or direct the group function. Sometimes this occurs as a form of competition with the leader. The dominant member may be unaware of his concern with power.

Doody, William M.

American psychiatrist. President, American Group Psychotherapy Association, 1947-1948.

Durkin, Helen E.

American psychologist and psychoanalyst who was a pioneer in group psychotherapy. Dr. Durkin worked with John Levy at the Brooklyn Child Guidance Center in 1937, treating children and their mothers in groups. Author of "Relationship Therapy Applied in a Children's Group" (*American Journal of Orthopsychiatry*, July 1939). She worked first with Lawson Lowrey, then with S. R. Slavson. She is a Senior Supervisor and Training Analyst, Postgraduate Center for Mental Health, New York. She recently has demonstrated the utility of general systems theory in group treatment. She is the Chairperson, American Group Psychotherapy Association Committee on the History of Group Therapy, as well as the Committee on General Systems Theory.

ego states

A term used by Eric Berne in transactional analysis. From his observations of patients' behavior and speech in groups, Berne developed the concept that all of us think, feel, and act from three basic positions which he called ego states and which he describes as "coherent systems of thought and feeling manifested by corresponding patterns of behavior." According to Berne, our personality is composed of three ego states which he calls Parent, Adult, and Child.

The Parent ego state is that part of our personality which

consists of the messages and slogans that we received from our parents when we were children. These messages he calls "parental tapes" because we go through life replaying them. Some of these messages are constructive and nurturing and some are destructive and based on prejudice. When we express them, they may be directed at ourselves or at others.

The Adult ego state, Berne states, is factual, rational, and straightforward and works best when it is realistic and not swayed by feelings.

According to Berne, the Child ego state thinks, feels, and responds just the way it did in childhood. The Child is spontaneous, impulsive, creative, and autonomous if it is a Free Child, or else it is an Adapted (submissive) or Rebellious Child.

emotional support (See stroke)

Members of a group and the therapist give emotional support to one another by the expression of feelings of understanding, encouragement, and hope.

encounter group therapy (See sensitivity training group; sensory experiential group)

A type of group therapy in which structured, planned activities and nonverbal exercises are carried out to give access to a patient's conflict areas. Emotional response is elicited usually through physical contact or group activities. A larger number of members (up to 20) can take part in an encounter group than in a psychoanalytic psychotherapy group, and the group runs a shorter series of sessions. Encounter groups are considered a group experience for emotional education.

Esalen Institute

An organization based in Big Sur, California, in which various group methods, particularly encounter group and gestalt therapy methods, are used to explore and expand the potential of intrapsychic and interpersonal behavior.

EST (Erhard Seminars Training)

Large group seminars devised by Werner Erhard in which participants are actively directed and led. The seminars usually take place on weekends. The aim is to enhance the view each participant has about his or her potential in life.

existential group psychotherapy

Group psychotherapy which emphasizes the here and now and the existential dilemma. Alienation and loneliness are feelings explored in depth and man's sense of being and its consequences in social terms. Genuine relationships between patients and the therapist take precedence over insight.

According to Hugh Mullan, existential group psychotherapy has no preconceived purpose but has for its goal authenticity and affirmation. Process is emphasized over content and immediate behavior over causal probings. Thus, the discussion can originate with either the therapist or patient, since it is based upon the here and now expression of the interactors and not upon a specific frame of reference.

existential position

Eric Berne in transactional analysis describes four existential positions:

1) "I'm O.K., You're O.K." reflects a positive attitude and means we can relate as autonomous equals. It is a winner's script.

2) "I'm O.K., You're not O.K." is the position of the person who thinks he is superior to everyone. Such persons, Berne says, start crusades against those they imagine are inferior. "At their worst," he says, "they are killers."

3) "I'm not O.K., You're O.K." categorizes the largest number of people. They feel inferior and think others are superior. They deprecate themselves and are depressed and neurotic. They have not received enough positive strokes.

4) "I'm not O.K., You're not O.K." is a position produced by too many negative strokes. It is a loser's script. A person in this position thinks he might as well commit suicide.

Ezriel, Henry

British psychiatrist and psychoanalyst who was associated with the Tavistock Clinic. Ezriel advocates defining transference in terms of the group structure. He advocates a three-level type of interpretation of group process: The group interacts as a whole to develop a defensive attitude to the therapist (the required relationship) so as to protect against anxieties (the avoided relationship) of a primitive nature (the catastrophic relationship). Group members unconsciously manipulate each other into the type of attitudes and relationships that will allow them to externalize unconscious inner object relationships.

Feder, Luis

Mexican psychologist who is a founder and former Institute Director, Mexican Psychoanalytic Association and founder and first President, Asociación Mexicana de Psicoterapia Analítica de Grupo; founder and President, Asociación Mexicana de Psicoterapia de Grupo y Psicología Colectiva; founder and first editor, *Cuadernos de Psicoanálisis*; first assistant editor for Latin America, *International Journal of Psychoanalysis* and the *Psychoanalytic Review*; Co-editor of the Journal, *COPAL* and editorial consultant, *Psychoanalytic Collection of London*; foreign member, London Group-Analytic Society; Co-chairman, First International Hand Shake of the AGPA, Mexico; currently President, Organizing Committee of the VIII International Congress of Group Psychotherapy in Mexico, August 1983. Dr. Feder has written many papers and chapters in books.

feedback

A term that refers to the responses that are elicited from other

o

members of the group by the discussion and behavior of an individual member. Feedback shows a group member the effect that his/her behavior has on others and gives him/her an understanding of himself or herself and an incentive to improve interpersonal relations.

Ferschtut, Guillermo
Argentinian psychiatrist and group psychotherapist following World War II. A founder and leader of the Argentinian Society of Group Psychotherapy. Editor, *Bulletin of the International Association of Group Psychotherapy.*

Fidler, J. W.
American psychiatrist. President, American Group Psychotherapy Association, 1972-1974. Secretary-Treasurer, International Association of Group Psychotherapy, 1977. Faculty, Rutgers Medical School.

Fieldsteel, Nina
American psychologist and psychoanalyst. Formerly head of Family Therapy Training Program and currently Senior Supervisor, Postgraduate Center for Mental Health, New York. Editor, *Group: Journal of the Eastern Group Psychotherapy Society,* 1976-1981. Author of many papers on group and family therapy.

field theory (See vector)
Kurt Lewin's concept taken from physics that views an individual's behavior as the end result of many forces in the complex energy field or life space that determines personality. Field theory is concerned with group dynamics. The theory holds that the components of a field (i.e., the members of the group) exist in dynamic interactions of the group to influence the individuals. This has implications for group therapy in terms of an individual changing the group and the power of the group to change each member.

filial psychotherapy

Psychotherapy in which parents are instructed how to help carry out the psychotherapy of their children. The group is composed of the parents of the children in therapy.

fishbowling (See group-on-group technique)

A technique in which a group in action is observed by another group. Sometimes a group divides in two and one group observes the other. Sometimes the staff or therapists form a group which is observed by a group of patients. The group being observed is in the "fishbowl."

focused exercise (See psychodrama)

A term used to refer to the use of psychodrama to help participants understand their feelings of anger and frustration. A male patient who is having trouble with his wife may be instructed to play out both his own role and the role of his wife. In the process of playing out both parts before the group, some of his own behavior and some of his wife's behavior become clear to him.

Foulkes, S. H. (1898-1976)

English psychiatrist and psychoanalyst. He was born Siegmund Heinrich Fuchs in Karlsruhe, Germany. He trained with Kurt Goldstein between 1928 and 1930 in psychoanalysis in Vienna. He practiced psychoanalysis in Frankfurt and emigrated to London in 1933. He first practiced group psychotherapy in Exeter, Devon, from 1940-1942, and his first paper on group psychotherapy was published in 1944. He transformed a military hospital into the first therapeutic community from 1942-1946. From 1946 on, he organized regular meetings with colleagues on group psychotherapy. In 1948, Foulkes published the book, *Introduction to Group-Analytic Psychotherapy*, Wm. Heineman, London. In 1952 he founded the Group-Analytic Society (London). With E. J. Anthony he published *Group Psychotherapy: The Psychoanalytic Approach*, Penguin, London, 1957. He was a distinguished pioneer who legitimized and expanded the use of group psychotherapy. A full bibliography is listed in *Group Therapy 1978: An Overview* (Wolberg, Aronson & Wolberg), Stratton, 1978.

fractionation of the group

The phenomenon in which the group breaks into subgroups and members act as individuals rather than as a group. It is a defensive resistance maneuver in which one or more members of the group detach themselves from the rest of the group in order to avoid becoming involved with the other patients.

Frank, Jerome

American psychiatrist and Professor Emeritus of Psychiatry, Johns Hopkins University School of Medicine. Conducted the first large-scale clinical research project on group psychotherapy with hospitalized patients and outpatients. Delineated recurrent patterns (roles) of patients' behavior in group therapy, notably the help-rejecting complainer, doctor's assistant and the self-righteous moralist. Contributed to the theory on cohesiveness and conflict in therapeutic groups. With Florence Powdermaker, authored the book, *Group Psychotherapy: Studies in Methodology of Research and Theory*, Harvard University Press, Cambridge, 1953.

free-floating discussion (See psychoanalytic group psychotherapy)

S. H. Foulkes' term for the group equivalent of free association. In this therapy a nondirective therapist gives a minimum of instructions and there are no set topics. Informality and spontaneous free association are encouraged. It undermines one of a psychoneurotic's strongest defensive positions, namely the desire to be led by an authority.

free group (See captive group)

A term used by Edward Pinney that refers to a group composed of individuals who are free to come to the group meeting at the office or institution where the group meeting is held. A free group is composed of patients who come from work or from their homes to a doctor's office for group meetings.

free-interaction group (See psychoanalytic group
        psychotherapy)
A group in which spontaneous and undirected reactions and responses occur. An analytic group that is based on the theory and practice of psychoanalysis is a type of free-interaction psychotherapy group.

Fried, Edrita (died 1981)
American psychologist and psychoanalyst who wrote extensively on the treatment of narcissistic patients in group therapy. She was a Senior Supervisor and Training Analyst in the Training Department and Group Therapy Department, Postgraduate Center for Mental Health, New York, and formerly Associate Professor of Psychiatry, Albert Einstein School of Medicine, New York. She wrote extensively, including, *The Ego in Love and Sexuality*, Grune and Stratton, New York, 1960; *Active/Passive: The Crucial Psychological Dimension*, Grune and Stratton, New York, 1970; and *The Courage to Change: From Insight to Self-innovation*, Brunner/Mazel, New York, 1980.

future projection
A technique in psychodrama in which a patient acts out his view of what he believes his future will be. The time, place, and person of the future projection may or may not be suggested by the director.

game
In encounter groups a game consists of a series of directed, planned activities involving bodily contact. They are designed to gain direct access to a patient's conflict areas and to release repressed emotions.

In transactional analysis a game is defined by Eric Berne as a "series of transactions with a con, a gimmick, a switch and a cross-up leading to a pay-off." Games are played out of awareness, and the series of transactions that make up the game ends in at least one player being hurt or put down and feeling badly. (See Eric Berne, *Games People Play*, Grove Press, New York, 1971).

Ganzarain, Ramon
American psychiatrist and psychoanalyst, who was the former President, Chilean Psychoanalytic Society and former Director, Chilean Psychoanalytic Institute. He has been a training, teaching, and supervising analyst in the Topeka Institute for Psychoanalysis since 1968 and the Director of the Group Psychotherapy Service of The Menninger Foundation, since 1978. He is the author of a number of papers on groups.

Garai, Selma
American art therapist associated with the Pratt Institute, also trained in analytic group therapy at the Postgraduate Center for Mental Health, New York.

gatekeeper
A role played by a group member who voluntarily tries to keep the group interaction going and who encourages other members to participate. He is distinguished from the "doctor's assistant" by his interest in order and protocol rather than group process.

general systems theory
Ludwig von Bertalanffy was the first to give the theory its name when in 1945 he published his concept of general systems theory. It grew out of his work in biology, in particular the theory of organismic biology and the theory of open systems. General systems theory recognizes that, while various systems differ in content, their general structure is similar. It sees all systems as part of an integrated hierarchy of levels, from sub-

atomic particles to whole societies.

In psychiatry, general systems theory focuses on man as a "system" ecologically suspended in multiple systems. It is based on the holistic nature of personality as compared to mechanistic, stimulus-response theories. Its aim is to integrate concepts of all the various levels of the systems that affect human behavior.

gestalt therapy

Gestalt therapy is a technique of making the patient aware of his unconscious conflicts and his unresolved problems through helping him become aware of his feelings as they occur in the "here and now."

Fritz Perls, the leading exponent of gestalt therapy, maintained that therapy can only be done in the now. The way a patient finds out about his feelings is to become aware of his tension, his heartbeat, his perspiration, the lump in his throat, the dryness in his mouth, his anger, frustration, or boredom. By focusing on his feelings in the here and now, he becomes aware of his unconscious conflicts and his unfinished business. "Awareness per se," Perls states, "by and of itself can be curative."

The word "gestalt" is taken from gestalt psychology. The gestalt is a configuration consisting of ground (general background) and figure (the figure that stands out from the background and that is seen as a pressing need or the satisfier of a need). The gestalt is open as long as ground and figure stand apart, and can be closed only when ground and figure are brought into relationship and incorporated into a single configuration.

An example of an unclosed gestalt would be a thirsty man walking in a desert. Water becomes his pressing need or the satisfier of his need. The gestalt remains open as long as he drinks no water. When he drinks the water, the gestalt is closed. Another example of an unclosed gestalt would be a person never having expressed the resentment he felt towards his father for not having talked to him. So long as he does nothing about it, the gestalt remains open.

According to Perls, the process of discovering long-standing, critical, open gestalts and closing them is a process of moving from neurosis to the authentic self.

Glatzer, Henriette T.

American psychologst and psychoanalyst who was the first (and only) woman President of the American Group Psychotherapy Association, 1976-1978. A pioneer in group psychotherapy, Dr. Glatzer worked in Brooklyn with John Levy and Helen Durkin when group psychotherapy was beginning to take embryonic form in the U.S. She has continued to teach, practice, and lead in the organizational aspects of the field. Training Analyst and Senior Supervisor, Training Department and Group Therapy Department, Postgraduate Center for Mental Health, New York.

going-around (See psychoanalysis of groups; structured interactional group psychotherapy)

Alexander Wolf's term for a procedure in psychoanalysis of groups in which each member takes a turn at free-associating about the next member.

When a good group rapport has developed out of the permissive atmosphere fostered by the free discussion of dreams, fantasies, and problems, the second stage of group analysis has been accomplished. At this point the therapist can then lead the group into the stage in which each member of the group freeassociates about the next member. Out of this "going-around" technique a number of unpremeditated inter-reactions occur. Each member is asked to say whatever comes into his head about another. He intuitively penetrates a resistant facade and identifies underlying attitudes. In a sense, patients are asked to become adjunct analysts. Making them active participants on a level with the therapists gives them reassuring status which is reinforced when they succeed in piercing the shell of resistance. Both the patient and the adjunct analyst benefit from the insight provided by "ringing the bell" or "hitting the target" in the course of this mutual examination. It is interesting to note that sometimes an untrained patient will uncover valuable repressed data that experts fail to bring to the surface.

Gomez, Angel G.

Puerto Rican psychiatrist who is Professor and Director of Programs on Community Psychiatry, Forensic Psychiatry, and Industrial Mental Health, Puerto Rico Institute of Psychiatry; Director, Consultation Center for Human Services; Visiting Professor, University of Puerto Rico School of Law; Coordinator of Programs in Criminal Justice and Juvenile Systems, Department of Addiction Services; Special Advisor to the Secretary, Department of Addiction Services; Special Consultant to Coalition of Spanish-Speaking Mental Health Organizations; Consultant, Institute del Hogar; National and Regional Consultant for Job Corps, U.S. Department of Labor; Consulting Editor, Hispanic Journal of Behavioral Sciences, University of California; President, American Society of Hispanic Psychiatrists; President, Committee on International Affairs, Puerto Rico Psychiatric Society; and Consultant to the Puerto Rican State Psychiatric Hospital and the Family Institute.

Dr. Gomez was also Chairman, Task Force on the Mental Health of the Spanish-Speaking People in the United States, American Psychiatric Association, 1971-1976, and Chairman, Committee on Spanish-Speaking Psychiatrists, American Psychiatric Association, 1976-1979.

Dr. Gomez is the author of many papers on group and family therapy, drug abuse, forensic and transcultural psychiatry.

gossip

A term used by A. G. Gomez referring to the talk that occurs between patients in a group when the group leader is absent.

Greenbaum, Henry

American psychiatrist and psychoanalyst who has published

widely on the topics of combined therapy and phases of group development.

group (See composition of a group)
A number of patients usually more than three and fewer than 12 brought together for psychotherapy. The optimum number for a therapy group is often said to be "more than the Graces (three) and fewer than the Muses (nine)."

group absolutism
A conviction that members of a group sometimes hold that their technique or style of psychotherapy is the only right one and that other ways of group procedure are inferior or unreasonable.

group acceptance
Acts or words of group members to a proposed new member of the group. Group acceptance establishes a new member's place in the group.

group-analytic psychotherapy (See psychoanalytic group psychotherapy)
S. H. Foulkes' term for the type of group psychotherapy that relies on psychoanalytic and psychodynamic principles and techniques.

group as mother
The concept of the group as mother is a transference reaction by the members of a therapy group to the group as a whole. The group is perceived as a benign, nurturing entity in ways that are analogous to a small child's perception of the good pre-oedipal mother.

group attractiveness (See cohesion; morale of a group)
The positive feelings that the members of the group feel for

each other and for the group as a whole. Related terms are group cohesion, group prestige, and group morale.

group balance (See composition of a group)

Group balance refers to the selection of patients for a group. There should be a combination of patients with enough similarity to provide communication and enough dissimilarity to promote discussion. The combination should result in a group that is likely to work together with a therapist to help one another rather than to resist change.

group bibliotherapy

Group bibliotherapy refers to the use of books, particularly in the treatment of institutionalized patients. Patients meet in groups that are larger than usual psychotherapy groups. The technique consists of the discussion of outside reading, the reading of books by the therapist and, in general, the use of books to promote verbal interchange.

group-centered group psychotherapy (See client-centered therapy)

A form of group psychotherapy derived from Carl Rogers' individual client-centered psychotherapy in which the members of the group, not the therapist, present the material for discussion. The therapist is supportive of the group but maintains a neutral position in the discussion.

Leonard Horwitz uses the term "group-centered group therapy" to refer to a form of group therapy in which the focus is on the reactions of each member toward the group as a whole.

group climate

The emotional atmosphere or predominant mood that prevails in a group is the group climate. A group may be generally pessimistic, optimistic, contentious, or harmonious.

group cohesion (See cohesion)

The emotional ties that hold a group together are referred to as cohesion. Libidinous aspects of patients' feelings are cited by R. D. Fairbairn as the source of cohesion. I. Yalom follows this formulation, but social psychologists give more importance to the cohesive power of a common goal or the threat of a common danger. The term "cohesion" also refers to the supportive behavior of a group in which patients work together and help one another.

group composition (See composition of a group)
This term refers to the selection of patients for a group. Sex, age, race, cultural, ethnic background, and psychopathology are taken into consideration when selection can be made from a large number of prospective patients.

Enough homogeneity is required to ensure effective communication and to "mirror" similar types of personality in the group. Enough heterogeneity is required to promote discussion. If all the patients were alike, less interactions would occur.

group contagion
Group contagion refers to the spread of an emotional tone or climate through a group. Emotions such as anger, fear, or mirth spread quickly in groups.

group contract (See contract)
The reality requirements for the members of a group include goals, attendance, punctuality, fees, meeting place, confidentiality, and manner of participation.

group counseling (See counseling group)
A type of group therapy in which advice or teaching is oriented toward a specific goal or difficulty in the present, through a problem-solving approach.

group culture (See group norm)
A term used to denote the style and manner of the group process. Standards of group behavior that are subscribed to by the group as a whole or that the group finds acceptable are

known as the group culture. Bion used this term specifically to refer to the group organization that develops and is able to reconcile a conflict between the desire of the group at any moment and the desire of an individual member.

group decision

A group conclusion reached by consensus or agreement. Kurt Lewin emphasized the importance of self-determination in a group and the relation between the group and an individual member of the group in arriving at a decision that involves the group as a whole.

group dream

A dream that occurs during the course of group psychotherapy in which the group processes are readily evident. Some patients dream of crowds or the lack of privacy, and some dream of the meeting place of the group sessions. Sometimes dream elements are recognized by the group members and result in significant progress in the therapeutic work.

group dynamics (See group process)

The interactions between the group and the therapist and between the members of the group. Since interpersonal relationships are at the heart of group psychotherapy, a full play of group dynamics and the psychodynamics of each group member advance the therapy and result in opportunity for behavioral change.

Kurt Lewin defined group dynamics as structures (or group configurations) that emerge when individuals are in constant interaction with one another. The individuals are interdependent parts of a larger whole, which differs from the sum of its parts.

group facilitator (See "assistant therapist")

A role played by a group member who directs or stimulates many of the interactions within the group. He may be playing the role to avoid discussing his own problems.

group "function"

When the group serves a purpose for a group member other than its treatment purpose, it is called a "function." Some patients use the group as a social gathering or try to make the group serve as a source of power and support for personal aims that are not related to the therapeutic work.

group growth (See phases of group development)

When the members of a group form a working therapeutic unit, the development is known as group growth. Group growth occurs when the individual members make themselves into a group that is able to go into action as a working alliance and do the work of mutual analysis necessary to achieve the therapeutic goals.

group history

Group history is a record of the episodes or events in a therapeutic group culture collectively known as the group history.

As used by Fernando D. Astigueta, M.D., at the Postgraduate Center for Mental Health, New York, group history is a written record of each session, similar to minutes, and read aloud at the beginning of each following session. The group history is used as a confrontational screen in the treatment of individuals with fragile ego structures because it maintains focus on the here and now, preventing disclosure of painful material from the personal history of each group member.

This technique increases the participants' awareness of their own interactions, their repetitive patterns of behavior as well as their assets and vulnerabilities. Therapeutic change is obtained through the medium of constructive feedback provided by both members and therapists.

group hypnotherapy

Therapeutic hypnosis carried out with groups of patients rather than with individual patients.

group locomotion

Group locomotion refers to the movement of a group toward the accomplishment of its tasks. Successful individual integration is the ideal outcome of group psychotherapy. Group pressures to conformity sometimes result from the group locomotion and may interfere with individual maturation.

group mind

A term devised by LeBon, a French sociologist, that refers to the functioning of the group as if all the members fused into one person, i.e., feeling, thinking, and behaving as one person. Members of the group behave in ways that are not characteristic of the individual but that represent the group as a whole. Bion also postulates a group mentality which has a uniformity, in contrast to the diversity of thought in the individual.

group mobility

The capacity of members of the group and the group as a whole to become spontaneous and expressive. The group becomes more mobile as the treatment program progresses satisfactorily.

group morale

Group morale is the degree of confidence with which the group proceeds toward its therapeutic goal.

group mother (See group as mother)

Group mother refers to the unconscious tendency of group members to view the group as a mothering, supporting, nurturing, and helping entity that facilitates survival.

The group as a whole is unconsciously perceived by its members as a need-gratifying maternal unit. These supportive and nurturing qualities relate to an early symbiotic stage of ego development preceding object constancy. According to object relations theorists, splitting of the mothering object into good and bad is a dominant mechanism associated with this concept. Consequently, while the group as an entity is perceived as the good pre-oedipal mother, the therapist and sometimes individual members can be experienced as the bad mother and become the target of hostile feelings.

group norm (See group culture)

The standards of behavior and attitude that a group finds acceptable to its members. Viewed as a microcosm of society, the group norm acts as a kind of social pressure alerting members to aspects of their behavior and attitude that are socially unacceptable although ego syntonic. It is one of the many varieties of rules of behavior and feeling, or do's and don'ts, that develop in the interactions of group members and become shared, perceived, and accepted as "the way we do things in our group." The group may adopt a norm that is not "socially acceptable" anywhere else, e.g., telling a member openly and frankly one's reactions to his or her behavior.

group-on-group technique (See fishbowling)

One group sits around another group. The inner group discusses a topic and the outer group later comments on and provides feedback on the group process of the inner group.

group pressure (See group strength)

The force exerted by a group on each of its members to conform to the group norm. The desires to be approved and to be accepted are the forces that operate within each individual. The forces that make group pressure effective are the desire of the members in the group to avoid exclusion or other sanctions and to enjoy a safe and familiar climate in which one knows the rules and feels secure and approved.

group progress

The forward movement of a group towards its goals, its course of action, and the techniques and methods by which a group approaches and works at problems and resolves conflicts.

group psychotherapy

A psychotherapeutic treatment in which a group of four to 12 patients meets regularly with one or two therapists for a period of time in sessions that usually last 90 minutes or more. The group discussions and the interactions of the members are utilized by the therapist to further self-understanding and to increase the capability of each patient to change.

Group psychotherapy is a form of psychotherapy where a trained practitioner (psychiatrist, clinical psychologist, or social worker) utilizes the emotional interactions of a small, carefully selected group to effect "repair" of personality problems. Patients are selected on the basis of diagnostic assessment and social, economic, and ethnic background. The group members know the psychotherapeutic purpose of the group and accept the group as a means of obtaining help in the modifications of their emotional difficulties.

group resistance

Group resistance is the avoidance or reluctance of the group as an entity to discuss relevant or pertinent material. Resistance may take the form of specific behavior such as silence, over-talkativeness, or playing out a group ritual. It may be reflected in the attitudes that interfere with the therapeutic work and the relationships of group members to one another. Group resistance is manifested by failure to observe the group contract.

group rigidity

The tendency of a group to continue stereotyped ritualized behavior to a degree that interferes with the therapeutic task.

group ritual

An activity of a group that occurs repeatedly, is participated in by most of the group, is generally acceptable to the group, but serves to avoid the expression of genuine feelings or thoughts. It is a form of group resistance that is mechanistic and repetitious and impedes progress towards the therapeutic goals.

group setting
The setting for a psychotherapy group requires adequate space and equipment for seating up to 12 people in a circular arrangement in an attractively but unobtrusively decorated room with adequate light and temperature regulation. Larger groups meet under special circumstances or for specific tasks.

group standards (See group norm)
The pattern of behavior approved by the group in their sessions and the manner and style of working that they adopt to attain their goals. The therapist plays an important part in the development of group standards.

group strength (See group pressure)
Group strength is the degree of pressure a group can exert on its members in its movement toward the group goals. This term can also refer to the capacity for work of the group members in their progress toward the therapeutic goals.

group systematic desensitization
A group treatment that uses behavior therapy to eliminate fear or anxiety. Members of the group learn to relax concerning a feared situation. Behavior therapy extends the relaxation to the entire group. Desensitization is based on the theory that relaxation responses are incompatible with anxiety responses.

group therapy for neuroses
Psychoanalytic group psychotherapy has as its aim the treatment of neurosis generally. The conflicts that result in anxiety can be analyzed and worked through by a thorough exploration of the resistances and transferences of the members using free discussion and dream material in the psychotherapy group.

group tradition
Over a period of time a treatment group acquires a growing importance to its members, because they recollect their common

experience in the group. The sum of these recollections is called the group tradition. The members' feeling toward the group tradition is a shared feeling that the behavior of the group is a live and meaningful identifying badge of the group and that membership in it has value and importance.

group values
Standards and traditions that are important to members of a group.

Gruen, Walter (1920-1980)
American psychologist who was Director of Group Psychotherapy, Rhode Island Hospital and Clinical Associate Professor of Psychiatry, Brown University Medical School. He also served on boards and as consultant to many professional institutions and organizations. His contributions to teaching and his publications on clinical and research issues in group psychotherapy were significant.

guidance group (See counseling group)
A psychotherapy group led by a didactic therapist. The group therapy in a guidance group is limited to a specific problem area. There is little or no exploration of the psyche or the genesis of the personalities of group members. The emphasis is on problem-solving of practical and behavioral issues.

Members of a guidance group receive didactic counseling rather than analysis or interpretation. Meetings may be scheduled at relatively greater intervals of time than the meetings of psychotherapy groups.

Hadden, Samuel B.
American psychiatrist who used a group educational approach for psychosomatic disorders in 1937, and did early work in the treatment of male homosexuals in homogeneous groups. In 1943 he used a therapy group as a means of educating medical students, interns and residents, and officers in the Armed Forces. Hadden's report on this technique is the first to appear in the

literature. He worked with Slavson, Hulse, and others to arrange the first International Congress of Group Psychotherapy. President, American Group Psychotherapy Association, 1948-1950. President, International Congress of Group Psychotherapy, 1980.

Hallowitz, Emanuel

American social worker. President, American Group Psychotherapy Association, 1970-1972. The first social worker to be elected President of the American Group Psychotherapy Association. He was initially trained by Slavson in New York City at the Jewish Board of Guardians and has taught for many years at the University of Chicago School of Social Work.

hallucinating psychodrama

A psychodrama technique in which the patient acts out the visions he sees or the hallucinating voices he hears. Leaders or directors of the psychodrama act out the phenomena described by the patient so that he may see aspects of his abnormal thinking put into action. The aim is to show the patient the unreality of his hallucinatory thinking.

Harrow, Martin

American psychologist. Director of Psychology, Michael Reese Hospital and Medical Center and Professor, Department of Psychiatry, University of Chicago. Author of many papers on group psychotherapy and multiple family therapy and of evaluative research in this area.

"helpful hannah"

The role played by a patient who confines his or her verbal participation in the group to discussion of the problems of others ostensibly to be of assistance to them but often in order to avoid looking at his or her own problems. Some group members may turn to the "helpful hannah" to avoid the work they should be doing themselves on their own problems.

help-rejecting complainer

The role played by a patient who solicits help, yet at every opportunity voices his dissatisfactions, lack of progress, and suffering. He or she rejects suggestions and recommendations for progress and relief and manages to find an objection to every effort made to help. He or she is usually a variant of a depressive-masochistic character disorder.

heterogeneous group

A heterogeneous group is made up of members with different demographic characteristics in contrast to a homogeneous group in which the patients are of the same sex, age, diagnostic category, and ethnic background. The limit to heterogeneity is the need for sufficient similarity to provide effective communication.

heterostasis in a group

When a new member is added or comes voluntarily to a group as a "replacement" of a member who left, a transitory disequilibrium is created. This imbalance arises from the loss of the "old" or nuclear member and the admission of the new one. Generally, reestablishment of the same equilibrium that existed before the change is not possible. Then, the group tends to strive toward a different or new equilibrium among its members (see homeostasis in a group).

hierarchy

The status of importance or power of each member of the group with respect to the other members and to the group as a whole.

homeostasis in a group

The tendency of a group to reach an equilibrium or balance among its members in terms of anxiety, activity, and progress. It is possible to evaluate a group's resistance to change and defensive structure in terms of the group homeostasis.

homogeneous group

A group made up of similar categories of members: the same sex, same general diagnostic category, same age range, and same socioeconomic and ethnic background.

A group may be homogeneous for age, diagnosis, or other category without necessarily being homogeneous for all categories. Homogeneity tends to promote group cohesion, but may limit the diversity of feedback that is seen with heterogeneous composition.

Horwitz, Leonard

American psychologist and psychoanalyst, Chief of Clinical Psychology, The Menninger Foundation. Formerly Director of Group Psychotherapy, The Menninger Foundation. Faculty, Topeka Institute of Psychoanalysis. Secretary, American Group Psychotherapy Association.

Hulse, Wilfred C.

American psychiatrist who advocated co-therapists in group psychotherapy of different sexes to "stimulate the creation of a milieu that repeats the family and society." In the early 1950s, he was head of the Group Therapy Department, Postgraduate Center for Mental Health, New York.

improvisation

A term used by Hannah Weiner and Zerka Moreno in psychodrama referring to the spontaneous acting-out of problems in interpersonal situations without previous planning or rehearsal.

inclusion phase (See stages of group therapy)

An early stage of a psychotherapy group in which the group members are concerned about belonging to the group, being identified with other patients in the group, and being accepted by them and by the therapist.

injunction (See script)

A term used in transactional analysis to describe powerful unconscious negative messages given by parents to their children. This becomes internalized in the Parent ego state, instructing the Child ego state. In response to these injunctions the child makes a choice called the early decision from which he develops a script or life plan.

intake groups

Groups in which new patients are seen before being placed in treatment, including group psychotherapy. The new patients are seen in a group and evaluated for further therapy. They can be given information and orientation to later psychiatric treatment.

Also known as vestibule, diagnostic, holding, or orientation-screening groups.

intellectualization

A process in group psychotherapy in which patients share, compare, and discuss specific objective knowledge. Intellectualization can be used as a defense to avoid discussion of the patient's concerns and feelings. Both intellect and emotions are necessary to develop insight. There can be a supportive as well as resistive function to intellectualization.

interaction

Reciprocal actions and reactions of group members among one another. Group interaction furthers the therapeutic aims of the group.

International Journal of Group Psychotherapy

The official publication of the American Group Psychotherapy Association. Wilfred C. Hulse and S. R. Slavson first suggested publication of a regular journal in 1948. The first issue of the Journal appeared in April 1951. S. R. Slavson was appointed as editor and continued for the next ten years. In 1961 Harris B. Peck became editor, in 1970 Saul Scheidlinger, and in 1981 Zanvel A. Liff. It is the leading journal in group therapy in the United States.

interpersonal skills group
A group for the purpose of helping group members improve their skills in social and interpersonal relationships. Attention is focused on communication and interpersonal contact techniques.

irrelevant action (See body language)
Also known as comfort movement, this apparently spontaneous movement such as stretching or scratching one's head communicates the nonparticipation of the individual in the interaction at the time. An irrelevant action communicates the sometimes deliberate message, "I'm not going to play in your game."

isolation
The group may ignore or snub a member or scapegoat him or her by assigning characteristics that other group members find unacceptable. One way this is done is by silence or changing the subject whenever the isolate member speaks. This avoidance is more noncommittal than overtly hostile as would be the case in "scapegoating."

isomorph
A general systems theory term referring to the basic structural features that are shared by all systems. For instance, individual and group psychodynamics are intrinsically similar and therefore isomorphic.

Johari's Window
The Johari Window is a device which describes how much of a person is known both to the self and others. It is a four-part square. Part 1 represents the part known to self and others (OPEN); Part 2 represents the part known to others but not self (BLIND); Part 3 represents the area known to self but not others

(HIDDEN); and Part 4 represents the part known to neither self nor others (UNKNOWN). The Johari Window was originated by Drs. Joseph Luft and Harry Ingham and takes its name from their first names: Joe and Harry.

Johnson, J. A., Jr.

American psychiatrist. Author of *Group Therapy: A Practical Approach*, McGraw-Hill, New York, 1967. Johnson's book describes a closed group in one of the few clearly documented examples of this kind of group.

joining resistances

A term introduced by Hyman Spotnitz as a paradoxical technique to get uncooperative persons to change by going along with their oppositionalism, e.g., a patient announces he will not come to the next session and is told by the group that maybe it is best he not come, even though he is required to come according to the rules of the group.

Jones, Maxwell

English psychiatrist who advanced the concept of the therapeutic community with prisoners and hospitalized patients, utilizing large groups as the main treatment category. Staff and patients participate in sharing decision-making affecting the treatment. Author of *The Therapeutic Community*, Basic Books, New York, 1953, and *Beyond the Therapeutic Community*, Yale University Press, New Haven and London, 1968.

Kadis, Asya L. (1901-1971)

American psychoanalyst who was a pioneering teacher of group psychotherapy and marital therapy at the Postgraduate Center for Mental Health in New York City. Editor with Jack D. Krasner, Charles Winick and S. H. Foulkes of, *A Practicum of Group Psychotherapy*, Harper & Row, New York, Evanston and London, 1963. She was Director of the Group Therapy Department, Postgraduate Center for Mental Health, 1955-1971. She had studied with Alfred Adler in Vienna and applied family concepts to analytic group therapy. She was an Assistant Professor of Psychiatry, Downstate Medical College, New York, and Supervisor of Psychotherapy, Post-doctoral Program, Adelphi University, New York.

Kibel, Howard D.

American psychiatrist, active for many years in the organizational life of the American Group Psychotherapy Association. He contributed extensively to the group psychotherapy literature, particularly in the area of inpatient treatment. Dr. Kibel is Director of Group Therapy, Cornell Medical Center, Westchester Division of New York Hospital, White Plains, New York.

Klapman, J. W.

American psychiatrist who began doing group psychotherapy during the 1940s. His book *Group Psychotherapy, Theory and Practice* was first published in 1946 and is still in print (Grune and Stratton, New York).

Kriegsfeld, Michael

American psychologist known for his contributions to gestalt techniques in group therapy.

Laqueur, H. Peter (1909-1979)

American psychiatrist. Born in Germany, raised and educated in Holland. Peter Laqueur received his M.D. from the University of Amsterdam. He first worked with his father, the discoverer of testosterone and Professor of Pharmacology at the University of Amsterdam. He became Director of Research for Organon Argentina S.R.L. in Buenos Aires, Argentina, in 1939.

Coming to New York City in 1947 he first worked at Mt. Sinai Hospital in Endocrinology, then in 1949 began a residency in psychiatry at Creedmoor State Hospital where he started his pioneer work with multiple family group therapy.

In 1968 Dr. Laqueur moved to Vermont State Hospital and continued his work with multiple family group therapy, developing videotape techniques. Dr. Laqueur retired in 1976.

Lazell, E. W.

American psychiatrist who was an early experimenter with the group treatment of mental patients. He wrote The Group Treatment of Dementia Praecox, *Psychoanal. Rev.*, 8:168-179, 1921.

leadership role

Leadership role refers to the attitude and behavior style of the leader who conducts a group. In social psychology there are three types of leaders: authoritarian, democratic, and laissez-faire. The role of the leader makes a strong impression on the group structure and function and is a major determinant of the character of the group.

This term also refers to a group member who assumes a leadership role by contributing knowledge, diminishing tension, or in some way facilitating the group functioning.

leapfrogging

A descriptive term coined by Donald Shaskan that refers to the situation in which a portion of the group members meet in alternate sessions so that continuity must be carried by the leader.

Lewin, Kurt (1890-1946) (See field theory)

German psychologist who came to the United States in 1933. Lewin studied group phenomena and coined the term "group dynamics" in 1939. Lewin was a group dynamist, not a psychotherapist. He viewed the group as an entity and thought of the individual in relation to the group in terms of concepts that he took from physics. In his field theory he thought of group members as forces in an electromagnetic field. Lewin participated in the early development of the National Training Laboratories in Bethel, Maine.

libido-binding activities

A term originated by S. R. Slavson referring to the behavior of children in connection with the objects and games that tie up their interest and energy.

Lieberman, Morton
American psychologist, who is Professor in the Department of Human Development, University of Chicago. Co-author with Dorothy Stock-Whitaker of *Psychotherapy Through the Group Process*, Atherton Press, New York, 1964, which introduces focal conflict theory and has remained an influential reference book. His research has covered life cycle development, the psychotherapy of older age groups, and the processes of encounter groups and self-help groups.

life skills group (See limited goal group)
A life skill group is a limited goal group whose aim is improving the social techniques of the participants. Members of such a group work on assertiveness training, anxiety management, career planning, and behavioral self-control to develop specific aspects of interpersonal relations in social situations.

life transition group (See crisis intervention group therapy)
A group planned to help the participants accommodate to changes in their life circumstances which occur naturally or at unexpected times.

Liff, Zanvel A.
American psychologist and psychoanalyst. Editor, International Journal of Group Psychotherapy; Director of Psychology, Training Analyst, Faculty Member and Senior Supervisor in Group Psychotherapy Department and Training Department, Postgraduate Center for Mental Health, New York. Editor of *The Leader in the Group*, Jason Aronson, New York, 1975. Author of many publications in group psychotherapy and related fields.

limited goal group (See self-help group; life skills group)
A therapy group for which specific and usually relatively quickly achieved goals are set up for the members.

limits for the group
The aims and goals must keep within the realistic constraints of the treatment situation. For example, the treatment of institutional patients is limited by the institutionalized setting. Once discharged and in a group of outpatients in a therapist's office, the aims and goals for which a patient may aspire are much greater.

Linden, Maurice
American psychiatrist. President, American Group Psychotherapy Association, 1960-1962. He did group therapy with obese patients.

Loeser, Lewis H.
American psychiatrist, who worked closely with S. R. Slavson. President, American Group Psychotherapy Association, 1950-1954.

Low, Abraham
American psychiatrist who was the major proponent of Recovery, a group-orientated rehabilitation program for former mental hospital patients.

maintenance leader (See "socio-emotional star")
The maintenance leader is a role played by a group member who is concerned with maintaining the morale or prevailing mood of the group. The role is positively characterized by optimism, encouragement, tension-relieving and active interventions to resolve conflicts in the group.

marathon group
A time-extended group. Usually psychotherapy groups meet for sessions of 90 minutes. Marathon groups meet in sessions that last several hours to several days. The sessions are interrupted only for sleep and food. The aim is to progress to the point where inhibitions are dropped and there is a free expression of emotions. Strong emotional reactions may occur in con-

nection with termination of the marathon group sessions. Theoretically the intensity of the session combines with fatigue to lower resistance.

Marsh, L. Cody

American psychiatrist who was an early experimenter with group treatment for hospitalized mental patients. He described the group treatment of the psychoses as the psychological equivalent of the religious revival meeting.

mattress-pounding

An encounter group exercise in which a member or members of a group vent hostility by pounding a mattress and usually accompany the pounding by shouting out feelings of rage. Subsequently, the other group members discuss their reactions with the mattress-pounders.

maximal expression

The fullest and clearest presentation of thoughts and feelings in psychodrama. It occurs as a rule in the psychodrama sequence of warm-up, action and post-action. The action itself usually presents the maximal expression of whatever activity is foremost. Abnormal thinking and perceptions may be displayed during maximal expression.

Mayo, Julia

American sociologist. Chief of Clinical Studies and Evaluation, St. Vincent's Hospital, and Clinical Asst. Professor in Psychiatry, New York Medical College. She does research on group therapy with manic-depressive patients.

McComb, Samuel

American minister, an associate of the Rector Elwood Worcester at the Emmanuel Church (Episcopal) in Boston in 1905, who helped Pratt begin his group treatment of tubercular patients and assisted Worcester in beginning his Health Conference. He is an author with Elwood Worcester and Isadore Coriat of *Med-*

icine and Religion: Moral Control of Nervous Disorder, Moffat-Yard, New York, 1908.

methods for group psychotherapy

According to Frank and Powdermaker, group psychotherapy techniques may be categorized as: 1) didactic; 2) therapeutic social groups; 3) repressive-inspirational; 4) psychodrama; and 5) free interaction groups. Reality-oriented integrative approaches may be included in the free-interaction category.

According to Giles Thomas, all group psychotherapy can be classified by the relative quantity of analytic or repressive-inspirational activity of the group.

milieu therapy (See therapeutic milieu)

Milieu therapy utilizes the whole treatment setting in a mental institution or hospital, particularly a hospital ward, as a therapeutic modality. The structure, the staff, the furnishing, and therapeutic activities are all coordinated to produce an atmosphere aimed at helping the patient resolve his conflicts.

Mintz, Elizabeth E.

American psychologist who has published widely in the field of group therapy, is the author of the book, *Marathon Groups: Reality and Symbol*, Appleton-Century-Crofts, New York, 1971, and has conducted workshops in group therapy techniques all over the United States and Europe.

mirroring

A term originated by S. H. Foulkes. Mirroring is a group process in which the patient sees his own behavior in the behavior of another. In a psychotherapy group two patients who have the same or similar problems reflect each other's behavior and give each other the opportunity to look at themselves objectively.

In this subtle process, an individual acquires greater awareness of himself through his interactions with others.

mirror reactions

Mirror reactions present another aspect of mirroring in group psychotherapy. A patient may see in the expressions and interactions of another group member a repressed part of his own personality.

mirror technique in psychodrama (See auxiliary ego)

A technique of psychodrama in which the patient is represented on stage by a therapist who becomes his "auxiliary ego." The auxiliary ego plays the role of the patient. The patient watches from the audience as though he were watching himself in a mirror.

The therapist acting as the auxiliary ego or mirror is also known as the "double."

modeling

The process in which a patient imitates consciously or unconsciously another group member or the group leader. In psychodrama the auxiliary ego may serve as a model for the patient.

morale of a group (See group attractiveness)

The positive feelings that the members of the group feel for each other and for the group as a whole. Related terms are cohesion, group prestige, and group morale.

Moreno, J. L. (1892-1974)

American psychiatrist who founded and developed psychodrama. Among his contributions was the "spontaneity theater" he founded in Vienna. After his emigration to the United States in 1927, he became a leader in the development of techniques used in group treatment. Moreno coined the term "group psychotherapy." He founded the Moreno Institute, which was a treatment and training center for psychodrama, in addition to organizing the International Group Psychotherapy Congress. He invented the sociogram which is a method of exploring affective binds in a group.

Mullan, Hugh

American psychiatrist who was President, American Group Psychotherapy Association, 1956-1958. In the field of group psychotherapy since 1948, Dr. Mullan is the author with Max Rosenbaum of the textbook, *Group Psychotherapy: Theory and Practice*, Free Press of Glencoe (Macmillan Co.), New York, 1962, and a subsequent edition. Dr. Mullan has been primarily interested in existential aspects of group psychotherapy.

multiple countertransference

A. G. Gomez's term referring to emotional reactions from the therapist to one or more group or family members.

multiple psychotherapy

When more than one therapist conducts group or individual psychotherapy, the treatment is called multiple psychotherapy. Co-therapy in psychotherapy is an example of multiple therapy.

multiple reactivity (See resonance)

The situation in which several group members react differently to the behavior of one group member.

multiple transference (See transference dilution)

Each group member reacts differently, because of transferential distortion, to every other member of the group as well as the therapist. In group therapy the transference reactions to the therapist are diluted or less intense than they would be in individual treatment where the transference is projected on the therapist alone.

mutual support

Group members agree with one another and encourage one another in the phenomenon known as mutual support. In the face of a common threat, such as mental illness, mutual support can lead to cohesion.

National Training Laboratories (N.T.L.)

Starting in 1947, the National Training Laboratories Institute for Applied Behavioral Science in Washington, D.C., began training professionals to conduct sensitivity or T-group training. This type of group is an experience-based form of learning to achieve knowledge in human relations, communication, and leadership skills. Kurt Lewin carried out the pioneer research in connection with group process and formed the theoretical basis for group work at the National Training Laboratories. Each summer since 1947, workshops are held at Bethel, a small town in west central Maine. Trainers who meet standards for election are appointed as Fellows or Associates of the Institute.

natural child

A term used in transactional analysis to indicate the spontaneous, autonomous, expressive primitive ego state of the Child that is not constrained by parental influence.

natural group

A group that comes about or has evolved among human beings without specific planning—for example, a family, clan, or religious group is known as a natural group. These groups serve a purpose in the maintenance of a society or civilization rather than as a means to effect change in the behavior of individual members.

Neiberg, Norman A.

American psychologist. President, American Group Psychotherapy Association, 1980-1981.

network density

A term created by Ross Speck in network therapy. Density is said to be high when people are closely related and know one another in close-knit networks. In loose-knit networks, where people are distant, density is low.

network therapy (See social network therapy)

A special type of large group therapy originated by Ross Speck.

nondirective group psychotherapy

A form of group psychotherapy in which the therapist functions as leader and permissively fosters free expression of thought and feelings in order to help members of the group to see themselves and others objectively. Dynamic interpretations and analysis are avoided. Theoretically, if group members see themselves clearly, they will go about self-improvement on their own initiative.

nonverbal communication (See body language)

Ways in which thoughts and feelings are communicated without speech. Bodily gestures, postures, and facial appearances are the most used methods of nonverbal communication. The scientific study of this field has been termed "kinesics."

nonverbal technique

In encounter groups, games and techniques involving bodily contact are used to convey feelings of trust and friendship. For example, several members of an encounter group may support, with their arms and hands, a member and lift him or her up to develop feelings of trust and confidence. Verbal expressions are bypassed in order to get directly at intrinsic basic feelings.

nude marathon (See encounter group therapy)

A prolonged group experience probably best described as an extended encounter group in which the participants are naked. Although it has the same duration as a regular marathon, the nudity is presumed to promote self-disclosure mentally as well as physically. Clothes are assumed to be defensive and to provide a protective facade, whereas naked bodies are considered less likely to be misleading in nonverbal communication.

objective countertransference

A broadened use of the countertransference responses of the analyst to the patient, not limited to the analyst's subjective distortions due to unresolved transferences. These responses in the analyst are due to the patient's attempting to induce or evoke them in the analyst through projective identification, so that the analyst corresponds to the patient's internalized object. These concepts were developed by Winnicott, Racker, Heimann, and Little.

A term used by Hyman Spotnitz to indicate the group analyst's conscious awareness of feelings induced in him by a group member and responded to openly by the analyst to express a limit of his tolerance.

object relations theory in group therapy (See Tavistock group)

Psychoanalytic theory derived from the formulations of Melanie Klein and developed by the British School (Bion, Fairbairn, Guntrip, Winnicott, etc.) which emphasizes the object-seeking propensity of the infant, instead of focusing solely on intrapsychic instinctual factors. The use of primitive defenses such as splitting and projective identification are important dynamics in this system.

In object relations theory emphasis is on the conflicts involving pre-oedipal drives. Issues of dependency and aggression are always related toward the important object, the pre-oedipal mother. Developmental arrest, object constancy, and the ability to deal with ambivalence are significant concepts. Object relations theory has been introduced into group therapy by Bion, Ezriel, Ganzarain, and Kernberg.

occupation group

The task or the purpose around which a group is brought together is its occupation. A social group has as its occupation the social pleasure of the participants. A work group or seminar group is a group for people with a specific occupation. The occupation acts as a barrier or framework to prevent disclosure of the emotional lives of the participants. The therapy group, since it is not an "occupational" group, allows freer expression of emotional and mental activity. A group based on occupation is not intended to be a therapy group.

O'Hearn, John J.
American psychiatrist. President, American Group Psychotherapy Association, 1974-1976.

open group
A psychotherapy group into which new members may be added and from which members may leave during the course of the group life is known as an open group. This is in contrast to a closed group where the number of members remains constant. S. R. Slavson referred to open groups as continuous groups.

openness
The ability of members of the group to express their thoughts and feelings freely and spontaneously. This is encouraged in the group, just as free association is encouraged in individual psychoanalysis.

Ormont, Louis
American psychologist who has demonstrated the importance of the contract and its relation to resistance in group psychotherapy. He worked closely with H. Spotnitz and used the paradigmatic approach to deal with resistance.

pairing (See basic assumption activity)
Pairing refers to two patients in a group becoming close to one another in a mutually defensive, supportive style. Pairing may result from characteristics particular to the two members or it may reflect a group resistance. As a collective phenomenon it can result from a variety of group conflicts.

W. R. Bion described pairing as one of the basic assumption activities in a group that employs the primitive, archaic belief that through sexual pairing a savior will be born, who will provide an omnipotent resolution to the conflict in the group. This form of thinking is probably related to primal scene fantasies and to Christian theology.

parataxic distortion
A term coined and used by Harry Stack Sullivan to denote distorted evaluations of another person that occur in interpersonal relations. It is distinguished from transference which was defined by Freud as due to a repetition compulsion of attitudes toward the parents during the oedipal period. Sullivan did not accept the libido theory as the motivating force, but considered the early nonsexual integration and coping with significant people as primary. By comparing one individual's evaluation of a person with others, one can come close to what is true, a process termed by Sullivan as consensual validation. Resolution of parataxic distortions thus becomes more readily apparent in group psychotherapy.

passive therapist
A therapist who does not initiate, structure, or direct the group discussions or activities. A passive attitude encourages emergence of so-called natural group culture which expresses the collective attitudes of the members. Passivity also fosters regression and projection of transferences. The term passive therapist is synonymous with nondirective therapist.

patty-cake exercise (See activity group therapy; encounter group therapy)
An encounter game similar to the palm-to-palm slapping game that children play.

peer identification
The conscious or unconscious feelings which prompt group members to identify with other members. This phenomenon

may provide support for group members who have poor self-esteem. Group members may admire certain qualities of other members and unconsciously imitate and identify with them. Negative identifications can also occur.

Perls, Fritz (1893-1970)

Frederick (Fritz) Salomon Perls was born in Berlin on July 8, 1893, and received his M.D. degree from Friedrich Wilhelm University. His analysis with Wilhelm Reich was interrupted by the advent of Hitler. Perls and his wife, Laura, are the co-founders of gestalt therapy, and with Paul Weiss and Elliott Shapiro established the first Gestalt Institute in New York in 1952. Perls went to Esalen at Big Sur, California, in 1966 and remained there for three years. Gestalt treatment is usually conducted in groups in a workshop setting where the therapeutic sessions are part of a total living experience for brief periods of time, such as weekends. The therapist's job is to catalyze awareness on the part of the patient.

Perls published many papers. Among his books are *Ego, Hunger, and Aggression*, Allen and Unwin, London, 1947, and Random House, New York, 1969; together with R. Hefferline and P. Goodman, *Gestalt Therapy*, Julian Press, New York, 1951, and Dell, New York, 1965; *Gestalt Therapy Verbatim*, Real People Press, Lafayette, California, 1969, and Bantam Books, New York, 1971; and *In and Out the Garbage Pail*, Real People Press, Lafayette, California, 1969. He died in Chicago on March 14, 1970.

personal growth laboratory (See sensitivity training group)

A group experience employing sensitivity training techniques which stresses the potential of the group members to become autonomous, creative, and spontaneous.

phases of group development (See stages of group therapy)

When a group is formed and its membership remains constant, specific attitudes develop at different periods of time which are shared by a majority of the membership. In the first few meetings the concerns of the group are mainly about organization and procedure. This is followed by a phase of constructive integration and mutual cooperation. A final phase is the termination phase.

H. Greenbaum compares the phases of group development to political structures of nations:

> *Phase I: Absolute Monarchy.* The therapist is seen by members as a feared and arbitrary leader; they project onto him omnipotence and power. Members prefer larger groups for support against intimidation by the leader.
>
> *Phase II: Constitutional Monarchy.* The therapist is seen as a benign and loving leader. The resistance takes on the form of wanting to be alone with the therapist and members become competitive with one another. Some patients wish to drop out or go into individual therapy.
>
> *Phase III: Republic.* The therapist is seen as an expert but noninterfering leader. The members are more cohesive and work more consistently on their problems. Conflict with the therapist and competition have diminished. New members can be introduced more easily.

phyloanalysis

The term used by Trigant Burrow to describe his group treatment. Burrow felt that the problems of the individual were reflections of the human race and that his formulations superseded Freud's emphasis on individual intrapsychic conflict.

A group method in which the focus of investigation was on the human condition with a de-emphasis of the individual group member. The term "phyloanalysis" reflected Burrow's interest in man's evolutionary and physiological status.

pillow-beating

An encounter group technique in which a group member pounds a pillow as an active way of releasing pent-up rage often accompanied by shouting in rhythm with the pillow-beating.

Pines, Malcolm

British psychiatrist and psychoanalyst. Director of Group Therapy (following Wilfred Bion) at the Tavistock Clinic, London; President, International Association of Group Therapy, 1980-1983. A colleague of S. H. Foulkes and Founder Member of the Institute of Group Analysis, London. Active in teaching group analytical psychotherapy at the Cassel Hospital and the Maudsley Hospital.

Pinney, Edward L., Jr.

American psychiatrist, who was introduced to group therapy in 1948 by George Naumburg, Jr., at Veterans Administration Hospital, Northport, New York. He taught group psychotherapy at the State University of New York, 1954-1968, Cornell University Medical College, Payne Whitney Clinic, New York, 1968-1978, New York University Medical Center, 1978-82. Author of *A First Group Psychotherapy Book*, Thomas, Springfield, Illinois, 1970, and numerous papers on group therapy.

pioneers in group psychotherapy

Historically, in the years before World War II there were few psychiatrists in this country who practiced group psychotherapy.

During World War II the large numbers of patients in military hospitals and rehabilitation centers together with the limited number of psychiatrists made the use of group techniques a necessity. It was discovered unexpectedly that the group exercised such a strong influence on the therapy of the individual that group therapy quickly became recognized as a potent and versatile treatment modality.

After the war the rapid and widespread practice of group psychotherapy was one of the most significant developments in the field of psychiatry.

Hence the war represents the dividing point between the pioneers who were individual theorists and the later group psychotherapists whose empirically based practices were suffused with modifications of psychoanalytic theory. Their work rested on the efficacy of the group as demonstrated during World War II.

The pioneers in group psychotherapy are (in historical order): Joseph Henry Pratt (1905); Rev. Elwood Worcester (1906); E. W. Lazell (1909); Alfred Adler (1918); Trigant Burrow (1927); J. L. Moreno (1930); L. Cody Marsh (1931); S. R. Slavson (1933); Lewis Wender (1936); Paul Schilder (1936); and Alexander Wolf (1938). (See individual entries.)

play group psychotherapy (See activity group therapy; S. R. Slavson)

Group psychotherapy for preschool children in which toys and play materials are used to help children express their feelings. Conflicts appear in the child's behavior at play and are clarified by comments from the other children or the therapist.

polarization

In an analytic group different patients may express strikingly opposite views or respond differently to the same stimuli. Polarization occurs when subgroups coalesce around opposing, extreme positions. Polarization may reflect certain basic tensions between group members, or it may result from collective frustrations toward a passive leader. These frustrations are displayed in the group matrix. While polarization sometimes reflects resistance, it often provides an opportunity for conflict resolution.

post-meeting or **post-session** (See alternate meeting)

Meeting of psychotherapy group members after the regularly scheduled group psychotherapy session. Such a meeting is sometimes held in the therapist's office, a nearby restaurant, or a member's home. The therapist is not as a rule present. In an alternate session this meeting offers additional therapy hours without the therapist. Material brought up in an alternate session is introduced into the regular session.

Powles, William E.

Canadian psychiatrist with Department of Psychiatry, Queens

University, Kingston, Ontario. Long active in the American Group Psychotherapy Association.

Pratt, Joseph H. (1872-1956)

Joseph Henry Pratt, a Boston internist, is generally regarded as the originator of group treatment in the United States. He modeled his classes on the Methodist Bible classes in Boston. Beginning with his "tuberculosis classes" (about 1905), Pratt pioneered group treatment to make sure that his patients followed his directions on rest, sleep, and diet.

preconscious

Material in the mind of each group member which is out of conscious awareness, yet which is accessible. All group members understand and agree with it once it is expressed.

pre-meeting session

A meeting of the members of a psychotherapy group before a regularly scheduled group psychotherapy session when the therapist is not present. Sometimes referred to as a warm-up session.

presentation

In group counseling, presentation is the term used by the group leader to orient a new member to the group. The leader explains the expectations, common problems, goals, and procedures of the counseling group to the prospective group member.

pressure cooker (See scapegoat)

Usually the term refers to the tension felt by a particular patient who is the object of intense discussion in the group, and who feels he is "in a pressure cooker." The therapist must be aware of the possibility of a "pressure cooker" developing for a patient who may be unfavorably affected by it.

The term "pressure cooker" must be differentiated from "scapegoat," in which an identified patient is not only the object of discussion, but also the object of displaced aggression. In scapegoating, the group members single out one individual and project negative attributes of themselves on to that one group member whom they make a target of aggression or scapegoat while they deny these same negative attributes in themselves.

primal therapy

A form of therapy originated by Janov, that involves the expression of the primal scream, which can be carried out in groups. Expressions of intense affect are encouraged, both physically (beating against pillows) and verbally. It is deemed therapeutic if the patient ultimately reexperiences the primal agony of birth.

primary group

The primary group consists of two or more persons in intimate face-to-face relationship, which has an enduring influence on the individual members, as opposed to a functional, work, or other group with which one has a limited association around a specific task. Typical primary groups are families and close friendships.

Group psychotherapy recreates the primary group and thus becomes a facsimile of the primary group.

process-centered group

A group in which the purpose is to study the reactions and interactions that occur between the members of the group. The dynamics and processes of the group itself are known as a process-centered group.

program (See script)

A term used in transactional analysis. The program is the internalized instruction of the patient, resulting from the parents having taught the child what he has to know in order to carry out his script.

projection (See transference)

A defense mechanism that operates unconsciously whereby one attributes to another person the attitudes and feelings of an important figure in one's early life, usually a parent or sibling. Sometimes one unconsciously attributes to others dissociated attitudes, usually negative, that one has oneself but that are emotionally unacceptable to the self. The other person is perceived and reacted to accordingly.

projective identification

This term refers to a defense mechanism based upon the fantasies of ridding one's self of an aspect of the self and the entry of that part into another person, in a way that controls the other person from within. It also involves an interpersonal interaction which promotes the fantasy of inhabiting and controlling another person. The influence is really expressed as an external pressure exerted by means of interpersonal interactions.

A later stage of projective identification involves the "psychological processing" of the projection by the recipient and the re-internalization of the modified projection by the projector. The recipient is the author of his own feelings; they are not "transplanted" from the projector. A new set of feelings may be so generated, which might involve the sense that the projected feelings can be lived with, can be acceptable.

The term was introduced by Melanie Klein and developed by the British Object Relations School (Bion, Segal, Rosenfeld, etc.). T. H. Ogden has published an excellent paper on the subject (*Int. J. Psycho-Anal.*, 60: 357-373, 1979).

Projective identification is a defense mechanism typical of the "schizo-paranoid position" of everybody's psychological development. It is therefore generally applicable to everyone. However, borderline, narcissistic, and psychotic patients may present more blatant examples of this defense mechanism since they are stuck at the schizo-paranoid position.

protagonist
In psychodrama the protagonist is the person who acts out on the stage his life or his view of the world to the group.

provocateur
The role of a group member who is frequently confronting or challenging and arousing hostility, frustration, or other responses in group members or the leader.

psychoanalysis of groups (See going-around)
Alexander Wolf's title for his technique of psychoanalytic group treatment which focuses on the individual in the group. The technique emphasizes dream interpretation, free association, and analysis of resistance, transference and countertransference. Wolf's method of "going-around" the group consists of each member taking a turn at free-associating about the member next to him.

psychoanalytic group psychotherapy (See free-floating discussion; free-interaction group)
Psychoanalytic group psychotherapy was developed successively by several psychoanalysts, notably Louis Wender, Paul Schilder, and Alexander Wolf in the United States and S. H. Foulkes in England. It uses the classic concepts and techniques of psychoanalysis, namely free association and analysis of dreams, transference, and resistance suitably modified for use in groups. It aims to produce a fundamental personality change in the members of the groups so they can resolve unconscious conflicts and maladaptive patterns and be able to function more effectively.

psychoanalytically oriented group psychotherapy
Group psychotherapy that relies on the theories and techniques of psychoanalysis. Recognition of unconscious conflict through overcoming resistances via interpretations from the therapist, other group members, or the patient himself. Each patient learns from listening to his own verbal productions, bod-

ily sensations, and nonverbal communications from himself and others in the group. Transferences are interpreted and new understandings worked through during the group sessions.

Clarification, confrontation, and interpretation, sometimes via formulations from the therapist, demonstrate to the patients the differences between the inner psychic reality and current reality. This is reinforced by consensual validation available in the treatment group.

In psychoanalytic group psychotherapy the leader is more active than in individual psychoanalytic treatment, but not directive or inspirational. Group meetings are held a minimum of once a week but may be held two or three times a week.

psychodrama (See role-playing; concretization of living)

A technique originated by J. L. Moreno in group psychotherapy in which the participants enact situations that are of emotional significance to them. One or more individuals take the role of themselves in the present or at some time in the past, or the role of another person, inanimate object, or animal.

They explore ideas and situations, verbally and nonverbally, while the rest of the group observes as members of the audience. The roles may be chosen or assigned. The enactment may involve situations that are hypothetical or real.

In order to gain a clearer understanding of self and others and enhance the involvement of the participants, various techniques are used, such as role reversal, doubling, or mirroring.

The psychodrama method provides an opportunity whereby the individual can express his anger, resentment, or old memories and through action discover a spontaneous self and new insights, developing courage and new approaches to living.

psychodrama director

The leader of a psychodrama session is known as the director, as in a stage production at a theater. He or she is simultaneously therapist, producer, and director. The patient is directed to put into action conflict and feeling, and responses are elicited from the audience, almost as a playwright would write for a Greek chorus in the theater. As therapist, he interprets the reactions and builds the interpretations into new actions, which clarify conflicts of the patient and the audience, for the patient's protagonist and the audience.

Moreno used Aristotle's *Poetics* as the basis of his system of treatment in group psychotherapy. Moreno also used Aristotelian techniques and mechanisms of catharsis for freeing long-repressed emotions.

reality-testing

Reality-testing refers to the ability of the individual to scrutinize his mental concepts to determine whether they come from internal sources or external stimuli. Ways of dealing with past emotional conflicts from childhood may prevent an individual from perceiving accurately and coping adequately with current environmental events. Hallucinations are an extreme example of a breakdown of reality-testing. The patient feels the hallucinatory sensations are coming from outside when they actually come from internal stimuli. In good reality-testing the individual has intact ego boundaries and current environmental factors are not distorted by past conflicts.

reality therapy

A kind of psychotherapeutic system developed by William Glasser, an American psychiatrist. The concepts of the immediate external reality, personal responsibility, and accountability together with the sense of right and wrong are emphasized. Patients are taken as they are and led to behave more in keeping with the requirements of the objective reality. Honesty is a prime concern in that it leads to freedom from conflicts with conscience. More attention is paid to behavior than to emotions or ideas in this kind of treatment. The duration of therapy varies.

reenactment

A term used in psychodrama to describe the acting-out of a past situation so that the patient may reexperience his mental reactions and reappraise his or her behavior.

reparenting

A transactional analysis technique in which a patient is regressed to a Child ego state and then supplied with a simulation of the missed parenting so that contaminations may be corrected. This technique is sometimes used in the treatment of schizophrenia.

repressive-inspirational group psychotherapy

At one time the popular conception of the mechanism of improvement in schizophrenia was "remission by repression." Early group psychotherapy in mental institutions was oriented along these lines. L. Cody Marsh, a former minister, treated large groups of schizophrenics utilizing group singing and lectures to inspire hope. Rev. Elwood Worcester also stated that the Protestant Church prayer meeting was the prototype for his type of repressive, inspirational group psychotherapy.

In repressive-inspirational group psychotherapy, the leader is active and directive. Group activities and lectures may be used by the leader. This type of approach is diametrically opposite to psychoanalytic group psychotherapy.

resistance in group psychotherapy

Resistance is the reluctance of a patient to participate in the therapeutic process. Resistance may be expressed as the inclination to avoid the development of a therapeutic contract or, after having agreed to a contract, not keeping to its terms. Talking too much or too little or sometimes remaining silent manifests resistance.

Interpreting various forms of resistance in the therapeutic process may result in the development of insight and personality change.

resonance

Resonance is the phenomenon observed by S. H. Foulkes in which the individual members of a therapy group tend to reverberate differently to any group event, each member according to the level of his psychosexual development.

The genetic theory of psychoanalysis supposes in every normal individual an orderly progress through certain stages of psychosexual development. When something interferes with the developing process, the individual may regress to an earlier stage of development or remain fixed at the level at which the interference occurs. The deep unconscious "frame of reference" is laid down in the first five years of life and predetermines associative responses thereafter.

This predetermination can be clearly seen in a therapeutic group where each member reacts differently to a common group event, such as the arrival of a new member, the holiday break of the therapist, or the behavior or emotion of any one person in the group. Each member reverberates or resonates to any group event according to the level at which he is "set," or regressed, or fixated.

review session (See going-around)
Kaplan and Sadock's term for a technique in their structured interactional group psychotherapy in which a specific group psychotherapy meeting is devoted to each member in turn, reviewing his goals and progress with the group.

role
In a psychotherapy group certain patients tend to play a part or role as actors do in a play. The patient will adopt a role and continue to play it steadily and recognizably during several group sessions. These stylized patterns of behavior are usually related to significant events in the patient's past life and are known as roles.

role allocation
The process in a group in which members of the group cooperate to put or hold a particular member of the group in a specific role, such as scapegoat.

role disorganization (See basic assumption activity)
Role disorganization refers to a kind of "identity diffusion"

that sometimes occurs in groups. With certain individuals regression in groups results in loss of coherency of self. The phenomenological counterpart of this internal state of disintegration of the sense of self is a disorganization of character patterns. The individual is lost in the group. He is uncertain what part to play. Interventions of other members of the group may help him reintegrate. At times, the bewildered disorganized self is a role that is used as a defense.

role-divided therapy

A prearranged strategy of co-therapy in which each co-therapist acts according to a special plan in the group session. For example, one therapist may become challenging to members of the group, while the other is soothing and supportive.

role flexibility

The ability of the therapist to take at various times the part of conciliator, investigator, or the role of one or more patients.

role lock

The phenomenon in which the role a patient plays both in the group and in life traps him in an unsatisfactory situation. Progress in self-fulfillment is made impossible by the role that the individual plays. The role becomes evident to the psychotherapy group; other members help the involved member to become aware of it and suggest alternative, better techniques of interpersonal relations.

role performer

The group member who spends a predominant part of his time playing an act of some type to achieve an effect rather than expressing his true, authentic feelings. He plays to the group members as an actor would play to an audience.

role-playing

In many group treatment modalities the therapist asks different members of the group to act the parts of important characters in their own lives or in the lives of other group members. For instance, a group member may act as the parent of another group member, an employer, or other authority figure to clarify feelings and attitudes apparently unexamined by the participants. New ways of dealing with persons significant in his life can be tried out in this way.

role reversal

A psychodrama technique in which one participant plays the role of the auxiliary ego of the patient, and the other participant plays the role of the first participant. This technique exposes distortions of interpersonal understanding and facilitates sensitivity and empathy.

roll and rock

An encounter group technique in which one member of the group stands with eyes closed within a circle of other group members who, as the member leans on them, pass him around the circle rolling him from member to member. Subsequently, he is placed lying on the floor and on his back, then lifted by the other members and rocked back and forth. Finally, he is placed again on the floor to conclude the physical part of the exercise. Group members discuss their reactions in terms of feelings of trust.

root group

A term attributed to S. H. Foulkes which refers to the original group in which the patient's conflicts arose, usually his family. Sometimes, as in conjoint family therapy, the root group is also the treatment group.

Rosenbaum, Max

American psychologist who has been an early practitioner in the field since the 1940s. Author with Hugh Mullan of *Group Psychotherapy: Theory and Practice*, Free Press of Glencoe, New York, 1962; and with Milton Berger of *Group Psychotherapy and Group Function*, Basic Books, New York, 1975. Clinical Professor,

Adelphi University Post-doctoral Program; Consultant, Harlem Valley Psychiatric Center; Editor, *Group Process*; Member of Editorial Advisory Board, *Group, Journal of Contemporary Psychology, International Library*, and others.

Rossello, Juan A.
Puerto Rican psychiatrist. Director, Mental Health Program for Puerto Rico, 1960-1973. Formerly Professor of Psychiatry and Head of Department of Psychiatry, University of Puerto Rico School of Medicine, 1958-1974. He is the author of several books in Spanish on group therapy.

rotation system (See going-around; structured interactional group psychotherapy)
The technique in which the therapist interviews the patients in rotation while the others in the group remain spectators.

"saboteur"
The role played by a group member who consciously or unconsciously undermines the progress and morale of others in the group.

Sager, Clifford J. (See Family Therapy Section)
American psychiatrist and psychoanalyst. President, American Group Psychotherapy Association, 1968-1970. An early worker in the field, Sager has in recent years added to the knowledge of marital and family therapy. His books include: *Progress in Group and Family Therapy* with Helen Singer Kaplan, Brunner/Mazel, New York, 1972; *Marriage Contracts and Couple Therapy*, Brunner/Mazel, New York, 1976; and *Intimate Partners* with B. Hunt, McGraw-Hill, New York, 1979. He is an editor of the *Journal of Sex and Marital Therapy*.

Satir, Virginia M. (See Family Therapy Section)
American social worker who worked with Gregory Bateson and Don D. Jackson at the Mental Research Institute in Palo

Alto, California. Virginia Satir started the first training program in family therapy in the United States. She was also the first director of residential training at the Esalen Institute in Big Sur, California. Publications include the books, *Conjoint Family Therapy*, Science and Behavior Books, Palo Alto, 1964, and *Peoplemaking*, Science and Behavior Books, Palo Alto, 1972.

scapegoat

The group member who is shunned, is not treated with respect, or is the object of aggression, onto whom is projected the negative feelings of others. The scapegoated member may be condemned or blamed for any or all the problems of the group. Occasionally the scapegoated member may stimulate this form of reaction through provocative behavior. The term is derived from the ancient religious practice of loading a goat with the sins and blame of the group and driving it off to rid the group of its guilt.

Scheidlinger, Saul

American psychologist who has been a long-time contributor to the field of group psychotherapy, and is Clinical Professor, Albert Einstein College of Medicine, New York. Scheidlinger was an early associate of S. R. Slavson. He is the former Editor, *International Journal of Group Psychotherapy* and currently (1982) President, *American Group Psychotherapy Association.*

Schilder, Paul (1886-1940)

American psychiatrist and psychoanalyst who was an early pioneer in group psychotherapy. He started psychoanalytic group psychotherapy at Bellevue Hospital in New York City in 1936. He also contributed to the literature on hypnosis and body image. (See Paul Schilder and group psychotherapy: The development of psychoanalytic group psychotherapy, *Psych. Quart.*, Vol. 50(2): 133-143, 1978; for an extensive review of his contributions, see Schilder, P., *Psychotherapy*, Norton, New York, 1938, extended, revised and arranged by Lauretta Bender, 1961.)

Schwartz, Emmanuel K. (1912-1973)

American psychologist and psychoanalyst who was Dean of Training, Postgraduate Center for Mental Health, New York, until his untimely death in 1973. He inspired an entire generation of group psychotherapists, colleagues, and students at the Postgraduate Center, which became a hub for the development of group therapy in the United States. With Alexander Wolf he wrote the books, *Psychoanalysis in Groups*, Grune and Stratton, New York, 1962, and *Beyond the Couch*, Science House, New York, 1970.

script (See decision)

According to Eric Berne's transactional analysis, the script is a life plan based on a decision made in early childhood, reinforced by the parents, justified by subsequent events, and culminating in a chosen alternative.

The script is developed unconsciously in early childhood and is based on the way the child was treated by his parents. The individual follows the script and continues to replay it in adult life. The script determines his or her style and the pattern of behavior. It is as if the unconscious script predetermines the real events of his or her life as well as the character and style of the ego.

self-analytic group

A group in which the participants are expected to do much self-scrutiny in a relatively short time. Examples of a self-analytic group are T-groups or sensitivity training groups. These groups are designed to teach group dynamics and interpersonal relations through examining the experience of group participation.

self-help group (See limited goal group)

A group of individuals sharing similar problems and goals who provide mutual assistance and meet without a trained professional leader. Examples are Alcoholics Anonymous, Overeaters Anonymous, and Alanon.

self-presentation (See psychodrama)

In psychodrama the patient portrays himself or herself and the significant figures in his or her life. In the course of acting out this self-presentation, the patient becomes aware of emotional reactions and becomes able to distinguish the realities from the distortions in thinking and feelings concerning people he depicts.

Semrad, Elvin

American psychiatrist who along with his followers made important contributions to the group literature on the treatment of psychotic patients in the later 1940s and early 1950s. He worked at Boston State Hospital where he trained many psychiatrists and influenced many people who treated chronic patients.

sensitivity training group (See personal growth laboratory; T-group)

A group that meets for a limited time to learn self-awareness and understand group processes. The focus is on the here and now and on experiential learning. It is based on Kurt Lewin's field theory of group dynamics and developed by the National Training Laboratories. This term has been applied by some to encounter groups.

sensory experiential group

A type of encounter group which explores the emotional and physical interactions of the participants. The emphasis is not on therapy or on group processes but on the experience of touching and physical encounter.

Shaskan, Donald A.

American psychiatrist who was President of the American Group Psychotherapy Association, 1964-1966. Dr. Shaskan was a pioneer group psychotherapist who worked at Bellevue Hospital with Paul Schilder in the 1930s. He has been recognized for his work in group psychotherapy with veterans of World War II and for his leadership in group psychotherapy in general.

short-term group therapy

Group psychotherapy in which the duration of the sessions is limited to six months or less. The therapist in this type of treatment must take up the issues related to termination from the very beginning of the sessions.

Slavson, S. R. (1890-1981)

American group therapist who, during the 1930s, experimented with a permissive method in group treatment with disturbed children in their latency period. This method he called activity group therapy. In 1943, he published *An Introduction to Group Therapy*, Commonwealth Fund, New York. He wrote many articles, reviews, books, and chapters in textbooks on group psychotherapy. He was the prime founding fellow and first President (1943-1945) of the American Group Psychotherapy Association and was the founder and editor (1951-60) of the *International Journal of Group Psychotherapy*.

Slipp, Samuel

American psychiatrist and psychoanalyst trained in group therapy by D. A. Shaskan and in family therapy by Virginia Satir and Don D. Jackson in California. Officer, Golden Gate Group Psychotherapy Association; President, Association of Medical Group Psychoanalysts; and Editor of the journal, *Groups*. On the editorial boards of *Family Process, International Journal of Psychoanalytic Psychotherapy*, and the *Journal of the American Academy of Psychoanalysis*. Director, Group and Family Therapy, New York University School of Medicine since 1968 and Medical Director, Postgraduate Center for Mental Health, New York, since 1979. He is the author of numerous articles in group and family therapy, psychotherapy research, and psychoanalysis, as well as the book, *Curative Factors in Dynamic Psychotherapy*, McGraw-Hill, New York, 1981.

social hunger
S. R. Slavson's term for the need of an individual to be part of a group and to be with other people.

socialization
The teaching of an individual, primarily by the family, to adapt and relate satisfactorily to other people in society.

socialization groups
Groups for patients who have been socially isolated by serious physical or mental illness or by other circumstances and who come together in a group for the purpose of being with other people to improve their social skills.

social network therapy
A type of group or family therapy devised by Ross Speck. In network therapy the group consists of all those who have been and are important in the designated patient's life. The number may be as few as 10 or 20 or as many as 200. The network or group is assembled and mobilized to reduce pathological dependency and to be effective in as many ways as possible to help the patient.

social therapy
A form of group therapy with psychiatric patients in which the aim is to improve interpersonal relations or social skills. Many forms of activity treatment, other than verbal group psychotherapy, function as social therapy—occupational therapy and recreational therapy are two examples.

sociodrama
J. L. Moreno's technique of using role-playing and dramatization to clarify social skills and enhance socially acceptable behavior.

"socio-emotional star" (See maintenance leader)

The role played by a group member who offers the emotional support that reduces tension and facilitates group cohesion.

sociogram

J. L. Moreno's diagrammatic representation of the relationships between members of a group. Individuals are represented by circles or squares connected by lines that vary in proportion to the degree of relatedness of the group members. Arrows and vectors show the direction of the preponderant positive feelings. This system reveals cliques, insiders, outsiders, central figures, and peripheral figures.

sociometry

J. L. Moreno's method of evaluating a group in terms of the expressed preferences and animosities that members of a group feel for one another. The most approved and admired member of a group reveals the status of the other members of the group. Sociometry involves a self-evaluation by each member. During the course of a group, the relatedness of each member changes so there are fewer contrasts in negative and positive feelings between group members.

Speck, Ross V. (See Family Therapy Section)

American psychiatrist with a background in psychoanalysis, family therapy, group psychotherapy, and community service therapy. Dr. Speck developed the theory and techniques of social network intervention in 1965 in Philadelphia. He is the author of *Family Network* (with Attneave), Pantheon, New York, 1973, and three other books. Dr. Speck is the author of 70 published papers and book chapters.

splitting of co-therapists (See splitting of the transference)

A phenomenon occuring in a group led by co-therapists in which a patient is unable to express ambivalence toward one or both of the therapists. The ambivalent feelings are split and projected so that one co-therapist becomes the object of negative feelings and the other receives the positive feelings. Splitting itself is a primitive defense in which others are seen as either all good or all bad.

splitting of the transference (See splitting of co-therapists)
Due to inability to integrate ambivalence, elements of the transference are split and projected separately onto several group members. For example, one member may receive the bad and another the good mother feelings.

Spotnitz, Hyman
American psychiatrist who has taught and written about group psychotherapy for many years. He is the originator of the paradigmatic approach which brings about change by going along with the patient's resistance (See paradoxical prescription in the Family Therapy Section). Author of *The Couch and The Circle*, Knopf, New York, 1961, and *Psychotherapy of Preoedipal Conditions*, Jason Aronson, New York, 1976.

stages of group therapy (See phases of group development)
Stages in the life of a group have been described as follows:

> Stage 1) *Forming*—the first 25 to 40 meetings during which the therapist develops a working alliance with the group.
> Stage 2) *Storming*—the next 10 to 15 meetings when authority, hostility, and group identity emerge as group issues.
> Stage 3) *Norming*—the period of mutual analysis.
> Stage 4) *Performing*—or working through which continues until the termination of the group.

Generally speaking, the terms, stages, and phases are used interchangeably; they are not used in ways that distinguish them clearly from one another. Various authors have described them in various ways. J. A. Johnson has described the stages of a closed group and H. Greenbaum has compared group stages to forms of political organizations.

In an open group where the number of members is subject to change, group phases or stages may shift. A later stage may change to an earlier stage when new group members are added or when other members leave. Termination has been suggested as the final stage of the group process.

Stein, Aaron
American psychiatrist who was President, American Group Psychotherapy Association, 1966-1968. He is Director of Group Therapy, Mt. Sinai School of Medicine of the City University of New York. Contributor of numerous papers to the group psychotherapy literature, Dr. Stein has made presentations on group psychotherapy regularly at the annual meetings of the American Psychiatric Association and the American Group Psychotherapy Association.

stroke (See script)
In transactional analysis, a unit of recognition or an expression of feeling given by one person to another. A stroke may be either positive or negative. It may be a physical action such as a pat on the back or a slap or a verbal expression of appreciation. The kind of strokes a child receives has a profound influence on whether he becomes a "winner" or a "loser." A negative stroke is called the "injunction" or "stopper."

structured group
A term S. R. Slavson used to designate a therapy group in which the members are selected with the aim and hope that they may have a maximal therapeutic effect on one another.

structured interactional group psychotherapy (See going-around; rotation system)
A technique in group psychotherapy developed by Harold Kaplan and Benjamin Sadock. The therapist structures the group so that at each session a different member of the group is the focus of attention of the therapist and the group. The whole

group and the therapist discuss the designated individual in rotation or turn.

subgroup

Attachment or alliance between certain members of a group. This alliance may be based on common or complementary characteristics and used for mutual support, or it may arise primarily to serve as resistance to the task of the larger group.

supportive group psychotherapy

Group psychotherapy which aims to maintain or enhance the self-esteem and the functional effectiveness of patients. Probing for unconscious conflicts and deep interpretations are not made, but bolstering of defensive structure is its aim. Although psychodynamic principles are used in supportive treatment, little attempt is made to achieve a fundamental personality change. Generally, supportive treatment is indicated for sicker patients whose defenses are brittle or shaky and whose self-esteem is low.

In supportive treatment, patients are taught better emotional control and ways of coping; the therapist is more directive, didactic, and inspirational.

Sutherland, J. D.

English psychiatrist and psychoanalyst who was the Medical Director at the Tavistock Clinic in its innovative post-World War II phase. He was an exponent of the British Object Relations School of psychoanalytic theory (particularly Fairbairn and Winnicott) and applied this approach to group psychotherapy. He was the former editor of the *International Journal of Psychoanalysis* and a consultant to the Menninger Clinic, Topeka, Kansas.

T-groups (See basic skills training)

The term "training group" is used to describe a form of experiential learning in a group where the emphasis is on the here and now and the group members are made aware of group process and the impact of their behavior on others. The object is self-awareness and realistic sensitivity toward others. The T-group was developed by the National Training Laboratories that developed out of the theoretical work of Kurt Lewin.

task leader (See "assistant therapist"; maintenance leader)
The role played by a group member who participates actively in the group, and facilitates the work of the group toward its goal by offering constructive advice, information and direction.

task-oriented group (See counseling group)
A group in which there is an explicit problem to be solved or a specific task to perform is known as a task-oriented group in contrast to a psychotherapy group where the emphasis is on the more general exploration of inner conflict and personality growth. Some of the same group processes and phenomena that occur in a treatment group that interfere with the group's work also can occur in a task-oriented group. Most of the social groupings found in everyday life are examples of a task-oriented group.

Tavistock group (See basic assumption activity)
A Tavistock study group follows the techniques that Bion and Ezriel used in their work at the Tavistock Clinic. The goal is to increase self-awareness and to understand group dynamics. In this self-analytic group, resistance to participation is seen in terms of Bion's thesis of basic assumption activity. Ezriel extended the Tavistock treatment method derived from Bion's work. This method emphasized interpretations of unconscious transference conflicts by the entire group to the therapist. The therapist assumes a nondirective and passive approach, frustrating the group members' need for structure. Interpretations by the therapist are to the group as a whole rather than of individual behavior. Regressive behavior to basic assumption activity may occur and be interpreted to the group members. The A. K. Rice Institute has extended this form of group treatment in the United States.

tele
The interpersonal reactions in psychodrama based on empathy and transference that stimulate cohesion of the group members.

termination
Termination is the final phase or stage of a psychotherapy group. In this phase of the treatment, the patient's work entails his separation from the group, mourning the loss and working through the unresolved residuals of previous separation experiences. An integration of the self occurs based on the preceding work done in the group treatment. Members become aware of the intra- and interpersonal processes that were developed in the group around termination. The use of this knowledge by the terminating patient and other group members results in self-determination and effective functioning.

terpsichore trance therapy
A kind of hypnotherapy originating in Brazil said to be based on ecstatic kinesthetic trance states accompanied by group dancing.

theatre of spontaneity (Stegreiftheater)
An early form of unrehearsed, improvised psychodrama originated by J. L. Moreno in Vienna.

therapeutic group activity
A term used mainly in inpatient and day hospitals. A group of patients engage in occupational therapy, recreational therapy, dance therapy, or similar activities. Therapeutically the group activity fosters social skills and promotes social contact and involvement, thereby deterring regression and mental deterioration.

therapeutic milieu
A specially structured environment in a mental institution or hospital where the therapist(s) and patients work together co-

operatively to facilitate therapeutic progress. Developed at Moorfields Hospital in England by S. H. Foulkes, it is an institutional treatment, usually residential, where emphasis is placed on group meetings and the common assets of the patients are utilized in the treatment process. Although the superficial structure is directive, the free expression of ideas in the group meetings is encouraged and acted on. Maxwell Jones also developed the therapeutic community where groups of patients and the entire staff meet together regularly to democratically share in problem-solving.

therapeutic social group

A group, such as Alcoholics Anonymous, that is organized to assist with specific problems. Such a task group is informally organized and arises in response to a socially recognized need. A therapeutic social group helps clarify problems, supports members' efforts to overcome difficulties or maintain a level of functioning, and in general works toward a broader social adjustment. It tends to be repressive and inspirational in nature.

therapeutic transaction

An interaction between patient and therapist or patient and patient aimed at improvement of functioning.

"therapist surrogate" (See "assistant therapist")

A role played by a group member in which he acts as co-therapist.

trainer

The leader of a sensitivity or T-group is referred to as a trainer rather than conductor or group leader of a psychotherapy group, functioning to teach group process through experiential learning. The trainer is certified by the National Training Laboratories to conduct T-groups but is not necessarily qualified to lead group psychotherapy.

transactional analysis (See Eric Berne)

A form of psychotherapy originated by Eric Berne in which the interactions that occur between people are seen in terms of the three ego states, namely Parent, Adult, and Child.

transactional group psychotherapy

The application of Eric Berne's transactional analysis to group psychotherapy. The aim of this therapy is to neutralize the negative effects of injunctions and other influences from parents and significant others so that the patients may free themselves to become autonomous and self-actualizing.

transference

The unconscious projection by one person onto another of the attitudes and feelings that he originally felt towards an important figure in his early life, usually a parent or a sibling. The patient perceives and experiences his relationship to others in the present according to these past relationships. Transference relationships may occur between a group member and the therapist or between group members, and may be negative (hostile) or positive (affectionate). The therapist helps the patient to understand his emotional problems with the original relationship and to show the patient that, while his emotional reactions may have been valid in the original relationship in the past, they are not realistic in the transference relationship in the present.

transference dilution

The term used for the phenomenon in group psychotherapy in which the transference feelings of a patient to the therapist are lessened in intensity as compared with the individual treatment situation. In group psychotherapy the transference feelings are distributed among the various members of the group, whereas in individual treatment the whole of the transference is projected upon the therapist. Group treatment may have a significant advantage for borderline patients whose transferences are intense and overwhelming, though fragile.

transference group

S. H. Foulkes' term for the fantasy group as opposed to the real psychotherapy group for each patient. The former is determined by the patient's transference reactions.

transference in group psychotherapy

Transference in group psychotherapy may be projected onto the therapist, other members of the group, the group as a whole, or groups more or less related to the treatment group. The resistance aspect of the transference is emphasized in treatment. Some transference phenomena, such as transference dilution, occur in group therapy.

transformation

A general systems theory term referring to the change in a system through the influence of another system or systems. In group psychotherapy the desired transformation in the patient system is a therapeutic transformation or change in the personality system of the patient.

translation

A term used by S. H. Foulkes to denote the process in which censored unconscious material is made conscious. This occurs in group analysis as well as in individual psychoanalysis. In a group every member of the group participates in this process with every other group member. Verbal and nonverbal communications, sophisticated clarification of mental processes, and "accidental" experiences in the group serve to facilitate this process.

transpersonal process

S. H. Foulkes' term for the collective interactions of a group. Foulkes considered that the transpersonal process was the basis for orientation, interpretation, and confrontation. He created the term "transpersonal process" to avoid what he saw as an arbitrary dichotomy between group and individual dynamics. He held that interactions between group members were more than "interpersonal" since they were embedded in a matrix of group interactions.

universalization (See consensual validation; reality-testing)

A phenomenon of psychotherapy groups in which patients become aware that their problems and mental operations are not unique but are common or "universal." This sharing of problems, solutions, and interests is supportive and provides a basis for lessened defensiveness and for learning and change.

valency

A concept taken from chemistry that refers to the tendency of an individual to join other individuals and combine with them in a group. Bion originated this term and applied it to the tendency of group members to join one another in basic assumption activity.

Vassiliou, George, and **Vassiliou, Vasso**

Greek psychiatrist (George) and psychologist (Vasso), who are group psychotherapists known for their presentation of the general systems approach to group psychotherapy.

vector (See field theory)

Term from physics used by Kurt Lewin to refer to the emotional forces felt by the group or by an individual in a group. One force may encounter a direct counter force, be deviated by another force, or combine with another force. Emotional forces are the social pressures that motivate therapeutic change in a group or therapeutic community and behave in ways that Lewin found similar to mechanical forces.

ventilation

The open verbal expression of the ideas and feelings that are usually repressed in social intercourse. This activity in group psychotherapy has a tension-relieving effect.

"war lover" (See "provocateur")
The role played by a group member who continually provokes ill feeling and conflict within the group. This patient hides fears and insecurities sometimes under an aggressive or provocative exterior and sometimes under a neutral exterior. At times he or she provokes the entire group to fight among themselves or with the therapist.

warm-up (See psychodrama)
The initial phase of any psychodrama session when the participants, the director, and the group prepare for action. The group discusses, selects, and understands the situations to be explored, and the director adds just enough definition to free the creative flow.

Wender, Louis
American psychiatrist who was a pioneer in the field of group psychotherapy. He has written many papers in group therapy and influenced other group therapists.

Whitaker, Dorothy Stock
American psychologist who was one of the pioneer researchers at Chicago (with Herbert Thelen) and who integrated Thomas French's focal conflict theory of psychoanalysis with group process. Co-author with Morton Lieberman of *Psychotherapy Through the Group Process*, Atherton Press, New York, 1964. Currently Professor of Social Administration, University of York, England.

Wolf, Alexander
American psychiatrist and psychoanalyst who was a pioneer in developing psychoanalytic group psychotherapy. He was influenced by Paul Schilder and Louis Wender. His 1949-50 article, The Psychoanalysis of Groups (*American Journal of Psychotherapy*, 3 and 4: 16-50), described parameters for group practice. First practiced group psychoanalysis in New York City in 1938. He was Director of Group Psychotherapy Rehabilitation Center, Fort Knox, KY, Feb.-Dec. 1943. He is on the faculty, a Senior Su-

pervisor and Training Analyst, Training Department and Group Therapy Department, Postgraduate Center for Mental Health, New York. He is on the Editorial Board of *The Journal of Psychoanalysis in Groups* (published by the Association of Medical Group Psychoanalysts). President, Association of Medical Group Psychoanalysts, 1959-1960. Received the first Wilfred C. Hulse Memorial Award for outstanding contributions to group therapy. Received the Adolph Meyer Award in 1951 from the Association for the Improvement of Mental Health "for contributions to psychoanalysis in groups." Honored by the publication in honor of his 35 years of outstanding teaching, supervision, writing, and clinical practice in *The Leader in the Group* (Z. A. Liff, ed., published by Jason Aronson, New York, 1975). Wrote many papers and books. Dr. Wolf at his first group in 1938 initiated the practice of "going around" and the "alternate sessions."

Worcester, Elwood

Rector of the Emmanuel Church (Episcopal) in Boston where J. H. Pratt began his tuberculosis classes in 1905. Worcester placed the resources of the church in support of Pratt's tuberculosis classes. In 1906 Worcester began his "Health Conference," a group treatment for nervous and mental illnesses.

Yalom, Irvin D.

American psychiatrist who is Director of Group Psychotherapy, Stanford University School of Medicine. He has contributed to the research literature in treatment groups. Dr. Yalom's work has been concerned with the interpersonal interaction in the here-and-now between members to help the individual understand and correct maladaptive interpersonal patterns. Author of the textbook, *The Theory and Practice of Group Psychotherapy*, Basic Books, New York, 1970, rev. ed., 1975, and other books and articles in professional journals.

Family Therapy Section

Ackerman Institute for Family Therapy
The clinic founded by Nathan W. Ackerman in New York in 1959 as The Family Institute. It was renamed after his death in 1971. The Institute is a major center in the eastern United States. Nathan W. Ackerman pioneered the development and acceptance of family therapy, using a psychoanalytic approach.

Ackerman, Nathan W. (1908-1971)
American psychiatrist and psychoanalyst, one of the pioneers of conjoint family therapy whose background was child psychiatry and psychoanalysis. Trained at Menninger's, he became a training analyst at Columbia Psychoanalytic Institute. He chaired the first meeting held on family diagnosis in 1955 at the American Orthopsychiatric Association and in 1959 founded the Family Institute (renamed, after his death, the Ackerman Institute for Family Therapy). He was the author of the first textbook of family therapy in 1958, *The Psychodynamics of Family Life: Diagnosis and Treatment of Family Relationships*, Basic Books, New York. In 1961 with Don Jackson he founded the journal *Family Process*. Ackerman's development of films of actual family therapy sessions contributed to the acceptance and widespread use

of family therapy as well as to the tradition of openness and use of audiovisual techniques in family therapy.

Adler, Alfred (1870-1937)

Austrian psychiatrist and psychoanalyst, one of the psychiatrists in Freud's early psychoanalytic circle who initiated the procedure of the same therapist seeing the parents and child(ren) during the same session, but separately. He was also a pioneer in group therapy and influenced the group work of Asya Kadis in the United States. His major contribution is individual psychology involving such concepts as the life-style, inferiority complex, masculine protest, and overcompensation.

adult-centered family

The interests and needs of the adults in the family are of most importance while responsiveness to the children is secondary. This was the common family structure in most traditional societies.

Alger, Ian

American psychiatrist and psychoanalyst who has pioneered the therapeutic use of videotape recordings in family therapy with Peter Hogan. He has taught family therapy at Albert Einstein School of Medicine and been responsible for the education of many family therapists. While he has been Program Chairman of the American Academy of Psychoanalysis, family therapy demonstrations and papers have appeared to a significant degree at meetings. He also was President, American Orthopsychiatric Association, 1979-1980.

American Association for Marriage and Family Therapy (AAMFT)

Organized by Lester Dearborn and Ernest Groves in 1942 as a professional organization which set standards for marriage counselors. It expanded in 1970 to include family therapists. The United States Department of Health, Education, and Welfare designated AAMFT to establish standards for certification of training programs in marriage and family therapy. In 1978, a 10-member Accreditation Commission was set up, which is aided by a 21-member Advisory Committee on Standards for Training and Education. Ten members of the latter are charter members of the American Family Therapy Association.

American Family Therapy Association (AFTA)

In 1977, following discussion at a meeting of the editorial board of *Family Process* in Cancun, Mexico, the American Family Therapy Association was born. Its first officers were Murray Bowen, President; John Spiegel, Vice-President; Gerald Berenson, Executive Vice-President; James Framo, Secretary; Geraldine Spark, Treasurer. Meetings are held yearly at various locations in the United States.

Andolfi, Maurizio

Italian psychiatrist who trained at the Albert Einstein College of Medicine and the Philadelphia Child Guidance Clinic. He is Director of the Family Therapy Institute of Rome, Italy, which includes Paolo Menghi, Anna Nicolò, and Carmine Saccu. The approach with families of schizophrenics that this group has developed starts with strategic family therapy and continues with structural family therapy. The family's initial phase of resistance to changing homeostasis and their need for control are used by the therapist in the service for change through strategic maneuvers. During the later phase when the family tends more to seek change, the transformational stage, structural techniques are used. He is also President of the Italian Society for Family Therapy in Rome, sponsored by the Institute. He has been published widely and is the editor, with Israel Zwerling, of *Dimensions of Family Therapy*, Guiford, New York, 1980.

Bateson, Gregory (1904-1981)

American cultural anthropologist and philosopher at Stanford University who had studied South Pacific tribes. Utilizing the theory of logical types (Whitehead and Russell) and general systems theory (von Bertalanffy), he contributed to developing the concept of the double bind in schizophrenia, along with others of the Palo Alto Group, whom he assembled—Jackson, Haley and Weakland. Bateson originated the term "metacommunication," which is a message about a message that provides a context, facilitating how the message is to be received and influencing the response of the receiver. Bateson was one of the theoretical giants in the field of family therapy. His writings include *Steps to an Ecology of Mind*, Ballantine, New York, 1972, and *Mind and Nature: A Necessary Unity*, Dutton, New York, 1979.

Bell, John E.

American psychologist who was one of the earliest pioneers to develop conjoint family therapy and the author of one of the first books published on the subject, *Family Group Therapy*, U.S. Government Printing Office, 1961. He was appointed Director of the Mental Research Institute in Palo Alto, California, after the death of Don D. Jackson in 1968 and continued in this position until 1973.

Bloch, Donald A.

American psychiatrist and psychoanalyst who is the Director of the Ackerman Institute for Family Therapy in New York and editor of the journal, *Family Process*, 1969-1982. He was a resident at Chestnut Lodge Sanitarium, where he studied with Frieda Fromm-Reichmann and Harry Stack Sullivan from 1948-1950.

He worked at the Clinical Center of the National Institute of Mental Health, a federal research hospital that opened in the early 1950s in Washington, D.C. There he worked with Fritz Redl and was the psychiatrist in charge of the children's psychiatric research unit at the hospital until 1953.

He first became associated with Nathan Ackerman in 1964 and became the director of the Ackerman Institute for Family Therapy in 1971, after Dr. Ackerman's death. He is the author of numerous papers and the book, *Techniques of Family Psychotherapy: A Primer*, Grune and Stratton, New York, 1973.

Bodin, Arthur M.

American psychologist who has been associated with the Mental Research Institute since 1965 and active in family research and in helping develop the Brief Therapy Center started in 1967 (with Weakland, Fisch and Watzlawick). He is the research associate and senior clinical psychologist of the Emergency Treatment Center which trains police to deal with family crisis, victims of assault, rape, child abuse, etc.

Boston Family Institute

Was founded in 1969, developing from a program begun at Boston State Hospital by Bunny S. and Frederick J. Duhl, Sandra Watanabe and David Kantor. In 1973 the Institute separated from the Boston State Hospital and established itself as an independent institution with its own quarters. The Duhls are its directors. David Kantor at that time left to establish the Cambridge Family Institute. The Boston Family Institute is known for the videotaped series "Perceptions," in which couples and families are interviewed by well-known therapists. In 1973 Bunny Duhl developed the "Interpersonal Vulnerability Contract" as a method to provide conditions of safety for risk-taking in learning and therapy contexts.

Boszormenyi-Nagy, Ivan (See contextual family therapy)

American psychiatrist who developed, at the Eastern Pennsylvania Psychiatric Institute, one of the important centers for training and research in family therapy. He edited with James Framo one of the early comprehensive volumes on treatment and research entitled, *Intensive Family Therapy*, Harper and Row, New York, 1965. His subsequent book, *Invisible Loyalties*, Harper and Row, New York, 1973, co-authored by Geraldine Spark, brought together psychoanalytic theory, systems theory, existential philosophy, dialectics, and ethics. Major concepts are the dynamics of loyalty, the ledger of merits (with indebtedness and entitlement through the generations), and the significance of relational factors. Contextual family therapy, which is a comprehensive relational approach integrating systems and individual dynamics, has been developed by Boszormenyi-Nagy and the Philadelphia Group. Boszormenyi-Nagy has employed philosophy, particularly ethics and the works of Hegel and Buber, as the foundation of his theories instead of physics, which tends to be dehumanized and mechanistic.

boundaries of the family

Boundaries serve to protect and enhance the differentiation and integrity of the 1) family as a whole (social system); 2) the subsystems of the family (i.e., parental, sibling, and generational subsystems); and 3) the individual family members.

Bowen, Murray (See family systems therapy)

American psychiatrist and psychoanalyst whose interest in working with families began during his training at the Menninger Clinic, 1946-1954. In 1954, he joined Lyman Wynne at the National Institute of Mental Health, where he studied schizophrenic patients who were hospitalized along with the mother originally, and later the father and siblings, too. He extended his original concepts on the mother-child symbiosis in schizophrenia to include the entire family in the concept of the "undifferentiated family ego mass."

Bowen then developed his concepts of the family projection processes, the scale of differentiation, the intergenerational transmission process (taking three generations to develop schizophrenia), triangles (triadic relations) in the family, and the importance of sibling position and family function. In 1959, Bowen left N.I.M.H. and joined the Department of Psychiatry of Georgetown University School of Medicine where he developed one of the most influential training programs of family therapy in the United States. One important technique was to return to one's family of origin to renegotiate one's relationship to further self-differentiation. Bowen also taught at the Medical College of Virginia in Richmond and in 1976 his staff moved into more spacious quarters at Georgetown University, the Family Center.

In 1977, Murray Bowen became the first President of the American Family Therapy Association.

Bowlby, John
English psychiatrist and psychoanalyst who was one of the first clinicians to explore and publish (in 1949) on conjoint family interviews. These were used as an aid to individual therapy and were conducted at the Tavistock Child Guidance Clinic in London.

Cassel Hospital
Psychiatric hospital in London (Richmond), England, whose Director was Thomas Maine and which admitted families as well as the patient for treatment. Various modes of treatment were used—community, group, family, and individual. The orientation was psychoanalytic. Malcolm Pines, currently the Director of Group Psychotherapy at the Tavistock Clinic, participated in this project.

centrifugal relational reality
A term devised by Ivan Boszormenyi-Nagy in contextual family therapy to describe an individual's reaching out and fulfilling the partners and children's emotional needs. It describes mature object relations.

centripetal relational reality
A term devised by Ivan Boszormenyi-Nagy in contextual family therapy to describe an individual's satisfying his own narcissistic needs from others. This is the motivation in Freudian instinct theory, where the individual sees others as sources of gratification for instinctual drives.

child-centered family
The parents give primary importance to responsiveness to the child's developmental needs and welfare, which in turn influences decision-making in the family.

collaborative therapy

A form of psychotherapy in which each spouse or member of the family is seen by a separate therapist. This has been the traditional form of treatment in child therapy, usually with the psychiatrist seeing the child and the social worker or psychologist seeing the mother. Periodically, the therapists confer for case conferences.

combined therapy

A patient is involved in family and individual psychotherapy by the same or different therapists. In marital therapy, the spouses may be in a couples group as well as being seen concurrently, individually or in conjoint marital therapy.

complementary family interaction

A form of family relationship in which members exhibit opposite behaviors. For example, the cheerfulness of one member might be accompanied by the depression of another.

concurrent therapy

A form of individual psychotherapy in which two or more members of the same family are treated simultaneously, but each member is seen separately by one therapist.

conflict resolution family therapy

The therapist helps the family learn to view conflictual interaction differently, and helps them apply alternate, new ways of problem-solving that better cope with conflict.

conjoint family therapy

An approach devised by Don Jackson in which the whole family is the therapeutic unit for treatment, and they meet as a group with the therapist in order to change family interaction. The objective is to change family processes that may contribute to the disorder in one or more of its members. Various theoretical approaches determine the therapeutic techniques. These include behavioral, paradoxical, strategic, psychoanalytic, systems, and structural approaches.

conjoint marital therapy
The marital partners are seen together by the therapist in order to study and change marital interaction.

consensus-sensitive
A term devised by David Reiss who noted a tendency for some families to have difficulty tolerating differences, and to strive toward rapid congruence or consensus of beliefs, feelings, and behavior. In his experimental work, Reiss found this to be a prominent mode of interaction in families of schizophrenic patients, but not restricted to such families.

contextual family therapy
A form of family treatment developed by Ivan Boszormenyi-Nagy which focuses not only on the individual's gratification of needs from others (the "centripetal" criteria of relationships, as described in Freudian motivational theory), but also on fulfilling the partner's emotional needs (the "centrifugal" aspect of relational reality which maintains the relationship). Systematic attention is paid to the impact of relationships on all partners. The concept of personal "entitlement" in contextual therapy describes the vested interest in and motivation for considering the reality of the centrifugal consequences of one's relationship. The intergenerational consequences are examined through the impact of parents on their children. People earn entitlement by mature human relationships and earn indebtedness from narcissistic exploitation of others. This is termed a "ledger of merits" by Boszormenyi-Nagy and Geraldine Spark in their book, *Invisible Loyalties*, Harper and Row, New York, 1973. The issue of loyalty, particularly in the child's efforts to help the parents, may result in "binding" (developmental arrest) or regression.

co-therapy in family therapy

Family treatment conducted by two therapists. This is frequently used as a training technique or with more disturbed families to prevent one therapist's being induced into the family system.

Detre, Thomas P.

American psychiatrist and one of the pioneers in working with multiple family therapy at Yale New Haven Hospital with hospitalized patients. He published the first paper describing this mode of treatment in 1961.

Dicks, Henry

English psychiatrist and psychoanalyst who was one of the first to set up a Family Psychiatric Unit, after World War II, at the Tavistock Clinic in England. Marital therapy was offered to couples referred from divorce courts.

disengagement/disengaged subsystem

A term devised by Salvador Minuchin to describe families that develop overly rigid boundaries around subsystems. Members of disengaged subsystems may function autonomously, lack feelings of loyalty and belonging and the ability to function interdependently or to request support when needed. In David Reiss' experimental work, a similar phenomenon was noted which he termed "distance sensitive," often found in families with a delinquent member.

divorce counseling

A form of professional help provided a couple who have decided to obtain a divorce. A therapist or counselor helps the couple handle the problems that arise during this period of separation and adjustment, particularly around the emotional impact on themselves and the children, as well as concrete issues.

divorce mediation

An alternative method to the traditional, legal adversarial divorce process. In mediation, a trained mediator, who may be a mental health professional or a lawyer, helps the couple problem solve by mediating differences to arrive at their own decisions regarding division of property, spouse maintenance, child custody, and support, as well as visitation rights. An attorney may also assist in this process to provide the framework of the law, but does not represent either member of the divorcing couple. The couple may then consult their own separate attorneys before filing for a separation agreement and divorce. Mediation takes into account, and helps the couple deal with, emotional issues around separation—anxiety, hostility, guilt, mourning, injury to self-esteem, etc.—to establish a reasonable mediating attitude. In this way, the divorcing couple is less likely to act out their emotional problems punitively on one another and their children around property and child custody issues. One of the pioneers in this field has been O. J. Coogler who is a lawyer and a marriage counselor. In California, mediation is mandated by law for divorce cases involving child custody. The traditional, legal adversarial divorce involves opposing attorneys, each representing one spouse, whose focus is on obtaining the best legal settlement for their client. Emotional issues are generally not taken into consideration.

double bind

A term originated by Gregory Bateson, Don Jackson, John Weakland, and Jay Haley, which describes a type of communication in families, initially considered to be pathogenic of schizophrenia. Now it is recognized as not necessarily pathogenic, but if so, not only of schizophrenia. There are two conflicting negative injunctions that are expressed at different levels (verbal and nonverbal) and must come from a person who has survival significance. In addition, the parent implies a threat of punishment for not complying to either contradictory message. Further parental injunctions prevent the victim from escaping the field or commenting (metacommunicating) on this no-win dilemma. The child or person is exposed to these double-bind messages repeatedly over a long period of time.

double bind over achievement

A term devised by Samuel Slipp to describe a form of family communication felt to be pathogenic of depressive disorders. The dominant parent communicates to the patient overt pressure for achievement, yet also gives a covert message to fail. The parent exploits the patient's success for his/her narcissistic self-enhancement. Because of the parent's jealousy and need to maintain control, the child's successes are not gratified and cannot be owned by the child. Thus, the patient feels trapped and cannot win, resulting in a negative cognitive set and feelings of helplessness. Compromise solutions by the patient are evolved to sustain some autonomy of the self, including difficulty making commitments, playing brinksmanship, self-defeating and/or oppositional behavior, or depression.

Duhl, Frederick J. and Bunny S.

Frederick Duhl, M. D., was one of the founders of the Boston Family Institute in 1969 and continued as Director after he left the Boston State Hospital in 1973. Bunny S. Duhl, Ed. D., graduated from BFI in 1971 and became codirector in 1977. They have developed an approach, "integrative family therapy," which takes into account the developing biologic and psychological individual, the evolutionary family system, and the broader contextual systems in accordance with general systems theory, and uses a wide variety of treatment techniques.

A map of the family system is devised which identifies its developmental stage, the ambiance and felt experience (or degree of jeopardy), openness to novelty and information access, the openness and form of boundaries, and the patterns of relating, and the "fit" of the individuals. The map of the individual members notes their cognitive stages and learning styles, vulnerabilities and defenses, core images, self-knowlege stage and communication skills, and the effects of these upon interpersonal and system transactions.

Known as educators in the field, the Duhls' writings reflect their attention to learning process in students as well as in clients. Bunny Duhl is developer of the Interpersonal Vulnerability Contract. Fred Duhl is developer of the Boston Family Chronological Chart and producer of the videotape series of family therapists, "Perceptions."

dysfunctional family

A family that cannot accommodate to and cope with stresses, such as those arising from changes in the life cycle of the family, usually involving addition or loss of a member. Boundaries between individual members are too loose, rigid, or distant, so that cooperation and support cannot occur. The family is not responsive to the developmental needs of its members. Homeostasis often (but not always) is sustained by one member being induced into being the identified patient, who overtly manifests symptoms.

dysfunctional marriage

A marital relationship lacking role complementarity, which may result in a dominant-submissive power relationship, coercion of one member, or the isolation of each member. Each strives for his or her own needs. There is poor conflict resolution, i.e., role induction or manipulation of others, avoidance of conflict or differences, triangulation of another member to form a coalition with, or expression of conflict through a scapegoat.

enmeshment

A term devised by Salvador Minuchin to describe the blurring of boundaries in a family. The differentiation of the family subsystems may be lost, resulting in loss of individual autonomy. (See also pseudomutuality; symbiotic survival pattern; undifferentiated family ego mass.)

Epstein, Nathan B.

American psychiatrist, psychoanalyst, and family researcher who contributed extensively to outcome studies of family therapy. He was influenced during analytic training by Abram Kardiner and Nathan Ackerman. He and his colleagues in Toronto rated change in the family by improvement in problem-solving ability, expression of affect, involvement, communication, role behavior, autonomy, methods to control behavior and family psychopathology. Currently, Epstein is Professor and Chairman of the Department of Psychiatry, Brown University Medical School, and Medical Director of Butler Hospital, Providence, Rhode Island. His method of treatment is termed problem-centered systems therapy of the family.

Erickson, Milton H. (1901-1980)
American hypnotist whose work with individuals formed much of the underpinnings for strategic family therapy. His ideas were used by Jay Haley as a basis for changing and influencing families.

experiential family therapy
A form of family therapy developed by Carl A. Whitaker which considers change as coming primarily from experiential learning and self-evaluation. Insight into genetic factors is not considered necessary for change; however, interactional insights related to the here and now of the treatment are valued. Co-therapy is encouraged, since it also provides a model or "meta-experience" for the family. Interpretations are most valuable when they are metaphorical and symbolically made about family relationships—using humor, teasing, fantasy, or free association to challenge the family's method of resolving stress.

extended family
A group of individuals consisting of the nuclear family (husband, wife, and children), as well as individuals related by ties of consanguinity. Extension of ties exists among parents and their children, grandchildren, and between siblings. In America the extended family has been common among rural and frontier societies, immigrants, as well as the very wealthy. Anthropologically, the term is restricted to two or more nuclear families affiliated by blood ties over at least three generations.

extended family therapy (See network family therapy; contextual family therapy; family systems therapy)

A form of family therapy that involves relatives related by blood ties as well as the nuclear family. For example, three generations may be present during the session, including grandparents, parents, and children.

family

The basic unit of society, characterized by two generations of persons bound together by marriage, blood, or adoption, who are emotionally dependent upon one another and responsible for their development, stability, and protection. Traditionally in Europe and North America, it includes two adults, one of each sex, living together in one household, who are in a legally recognized relationship (marriage by license or common-law acceptance), with one or more children who are first-degree biologically related or adopted. The family serves as the basic unit of socialization, to teach cultural values and facilitate adaptation to society.

In a single parent family, only one person serves in the maternal or paternal role to one or more children. Due to the high death rate in the past and the high divorce rate in the present, the number of single parent families has always been high.

family art therapy

A form of therapy employing art techniques conducted with the whole family to observe how the family unit operates and to facilitate the process of family therapy. The use of art materials and the use of verbal techniques are considered to be mutually facilitating on an ongoing basis.

family boundary marker

A term devised by Salvador Minuchin whereby the therapist joins with one subsystem of the family and excludes others during sessions of the entire family to differentiate boundaries.

family-centered family
There is a strong emphasis on the importance of the whole family as a unit, and individuals are submerged to the needs and functions of the family group.

family climate
Each family has a general emotional atmosphere or tone. At times the emotional climate may be difficult to perceive as it truly exists, because of a facade created for others.

family developmental tasks
At each stage in the life cycle of the family, there are certain role expectations of its members sanctioned by society. The successful achievement of these norms leads to satisfactions, equilibrium of the family, and success with later tasks. Failure leads to distress in the family, disapproval and sanctions by society, and emotional problems with later developmental tasks. For example, during infancy the mother seeks to fulfill the child's symbiotic needs for merging, but during adolescence the family needs to allow for individuation and separation.

family dyad
The relationship between any two family members, e.g., father-mother, father-son, mother-son, brother-sister.

family dynamics
The intrapsychic, interpersonal, and family-as-a-whole patterns operating in the family system, such as thoughts, feelings, and behavior, conscious or unconscious, in which two or more members of the family consistently engage, as well as the attitudes and emotional climate which the whole family maintains as the framework for its relationships.

family homeostasis
A theory postulated by Don Jackson that the family is a unit or organization having an internal and ongoing, interactional

process and rule structure to maintain a relative constancy or balance of relationships. There is resistance to change in relationships, and this is achieved by an error-activated feedback system. This balance in relationships may require one individual to be the identified patient, who is manifestly disturbed, in order to preserve the functional integrity of other members of the family. Family homeostasis is an analogue of physiologic homeostasis as formulated earlier by Walter Cannon. Morphostasis, in general systems theory, is a synonym of homeostasis that more clearly places the emphasis on tendencies to maintain a "steady state" and lack of change. Nathan Ackerman also spoke of family homeo*dynamic* processes to indicate that internal changes constantly take place, not *stasis*, even though the family as a *system* remains relatively the same.

family map
An organizational schematic representation used in structural family therapy, which permits the therapist to develop hypotheses about areas that may be dysfunctional in a family and helps to determine therapeutic goals.

family myths
Refers to a set of beliefs based on kernels of historic reality but elaborated and shared by all family members that help determine and shape the rules governing relationships in the family. These beliefs go unchallenged by everyone involved, despite partial distortions of current reality. All families have myths as a prerequisite to their functioning as social units having continuity. When myths and current reality become highly discrepant, the existence of the myths is more readily apparent, but most family myths are smoothly contributory to "healthy" family functioning.

family of origin
The family into which a person is born or adopted.

family of procreation
The family formed by marriage and in which the person becomes a parent.

family process
The totality of the transactions in the family.

Family Process Journal
The first journal published in family therapy which was founded in 1961 by Don D. Jackson and Nathan W. Ackerman as a collaborative effort between the Mental Research Institute in Palo Alto, California, and The Family Institute of New York (renamed the Ackerman Institute for Family Therapy) in New York City. Jay Haley was its first editor until 1969, when Donald Bloch assumed editorship. Carlos E. Sluzki becomes editor in 1983. This is a multidisciplinary journal of family study, research, and treatment that is published quarterly. Its Editorial Board and Board of Advisory Editors encompass most of the current leadership in the field of family therapy and research.

family projection process
The process by which parental problems, conflicts, or internalized images are projected onto children and/or the spouse. Murray Bowen traces the intergenerational transmission of patterns in the family by this process. Lyman Wynne, Roger Shapiro, and Samuel Slipp use projection-identification as the primary mode by which pathology is induced in patients.

family ritual
A therapeutic technique employed by the Milan Group of Selvini Palazzoli that prescribes an act or group of acts that family members perform at a specific time, place, for a number of times which tend to change the family system of rules.

family role
Family members *assume* a particular position and perform the

associated role, containing certain rights and obligations. For example, a man may be father, husband, breadwinner, lover, etc. Some roles are shared or exchanged at times. Conflict can occur when several members of the family perceive a given role differently, i.e., a husband and wife may see the role of wife differently. Some family roles are *assigned*, such as go-between, savior, scapegoat, etc., which may or may not be pathogenic.

family sculpting

An experiential technique originated by Virginia Satir and used in family therapy, in which the members are asked to make a nonverbal statement about themselves and their family by positioning themselves through posture, gesture, and facial expression to form a tableau of their relationships.

family structure

A term used to describe the functional organization of the family that determines the manner in which members interact and communicate.

family system

A network of transactions that sustains both homeostasis (morphostasis) and change (morphogenesis) and, *secondarily*, helps determine and is determined by individual behavior of family members. Murray Bowen's form of family therapy focuses on understanding these networks and has been termed "systems approach." His use of this term differs from the broader and more fully conceptualized concept of systems developed by Ludwig von Bertalanffy in general systems theory, by Talcott Parsons in family sociology, and by John Spiegel in the early 1950s.

family systems theory

Family systems theory has also been used synonomously with Murray Bowen's approach to family therapy. Bowen examines family structure and function of various systems: between the generations, within the family in terms of triangles and alliances, as well as the level of differentiation of its individual members. Each subsystem of the family is related to another and determines the behavior and functioning of its members. Patterns of transactions are repeated through the generations. Bowen considers at least three generations of increasing lack of differentiation of its members are necessary to produce a schizophrenic patient. (See also multigenerational transmission process; symbiotic survival pattern.)

family systems therapy (Bowenian family therapy)

One of the leading forms of family therapy whose theory and practice were developed by Murray Bowen. The theory is based on six major concepts: 1) triangles—triadic relations with two inside and one outside positions; 2) family emotional process—distancing, conflict, one spouse can diminish functioning, or the couple can develop a common concern for a child; 3) family projection process—how undifferentiation is transmitted; 4) scale of differentiation of individuals—lower-level families are dominated by emotional and group forces; 5) multigenerational transmission process—investigating three generations' patterns; 6) emotional cutoff—to deal with unresolved fusion; 7) sibling position—determines personality functioning, especially the assumption of responsibility; and 8) societal emotional process—influences the family in terms of togetherness or individuality. Bowenian therapy investigates the extended family, looking for repetitious patterns through the generations.

Renegotiating unresolved issues by the spouse with his or her own family of origin is stressed to increase differentiation of the self.

family therapy

A form of treatment of the whole family as a group together by one or two therapists. Individual pathology in one member is seen as a reflection of wider pathology in the family system. The family unit thus becomes the unit treated and changing the family interaction is seen as changing the identified member's pathology.

Flugel, J. C. (1884-1955)

An early psychoanalyst whose book *The Psychoanalytic Study of the Family*, Hogarth, London, 1921, pioneered the exploration of the family in the etiology and maintenance of neurosis.

Framo, James

American psychologist who has been an early and prolific contributor to the literature, and educator of marital and family therapy. He worked with Ivan Boszormenyi-Nagy at the Eastern Pennsylvania Psychiatric Institute resulting in their editing the book, *Intensive Family Therapy*, Harper and Row, New York, 1965. Framo is currently Professor, Department of Psychology, Temple University in Philadelphia and has consulted on short-term approaches to marital therapy. Since children who may be disturbed come from disturbed marriages, the focus is on treating the marital couple. Framo has been influenced by the object relations theory of Fairbairn and marital interaction theory of Dicks. Like Bowen, Framo encourages adults to return to their family of origin to resolve conflict and renegotiate their relationships. He is also the author of the book, *Family Interaction, A Dialogue Between Family Researchers and Family Therapists*, Springer, New York, 1972.

Freud, Sigmund (1856-1939)

Austrian psychiatrist and the father of psychoanalysis. Freud was one of the first psychiatrists to study and note the influence of the family on the development of symptomatology in the patient. In his case history of Little Hans, Freud worked with the father to enable the son to test out and work through the oedipal conflict and castration fears leading to resolution of the son's phobia. Freud is known to have explored concurrent, simultaneous analyses with James and Alex Strachey, as well as with another family.

Friedman, Leonard J.

American psychiatrist and psychoanalyst who organized the Society of Family Therapy and Research and was one of the originators of the Cambridge Family Institute, Cambridge, Massachusetts. He is Assistant Clinical Professor of Psychiatry at Harvard Medical School. Friedman has attempted to bring together psychoanalytic (object relations) theory and family systems theory. He is the author of papers in the field and co-author with John K. Pearce of the book, *Family Therapy: Combining Psychodynamics and Family Systems Approaches*, Grune and Stratton, New York, 1980.

functional family
A family in which there is complementarity between its members, with mutual accommodation to each other's needs, clear and flexible boundaries between individuals, and ability to resolve conflict and create change in accord with the family's life cycle.

general systems theory (See systems theory)
General systems theory was formulated by Ludwig von Bertalanffy in 1945 as a general scientific theory whose principles are valid for living as well as nonliving systems. Systems are seen as open, with various levels or subsystems standing in relation to one another. The aim of general systems theory is to find general isomorphisms in systems and to look for organization or structure of the various subsystems. Each subsystem has a boundary and a degree of autonomy, but is interactive with and dependent upon general control by the suprasystem of which it is a part. Feedback loops adjust the functioning of the system to maintain general continuity, function and structure (negative feedback—morphostasis). Yet the system is open enough to permit growth and development within limits (positive feedback—morphogenesis). Family homeostasis is an example of morphostasis which was devised by Don D. Jackson. General systems theory finds expression in many theories and practices of family therapy. The work of John P. Spiegel, which covers the transactional field of universe, culture, society, group,

psyche, and soma comes closest, in encompassing the greatest breadth, to general systems theory.

generational boundary

The boundary between parents and children who are a generation apart. Theodore Lidz noted that disruption of this boundary occurred in families with a schizophrenic child.

genogram

A schematic diagram of the family relationship system based on the genetic tree, usually involving two or three generations. Squares are used to represent men and circles to indicate women. These are tied together with a horizontal line to indicate marriage (the date of marriage may be entered here) and vertical lines drawn down from the horizontal, with the appropriate square or circle to indicate children and their sex. The ages of these individuals may be entered in the square or circle. The families of origin may then be drawn in with parents and siblings of each spouse. Death of a member is indicated by placing a cross over the square or box. Other important events may be listed as well as indications of patterns of alliance and conflict; the former may be indicated by a straight line drawn between the members and the latter by a curvy line. Bowenian therapists use the genogram to determine triangles and may use it therapeutically in the sessions.

go-between (go-between therapy)

A term used by Gerald Zuk whereby the therapist in family therapy takes the role of mediator between two people in a conflict, trying to change a pathogenic relationship by focusing on issues for the two to negotiate. Cessation of conflict can occur when there is a change in the positions of the principals or a redefinition of the conflict.

A term employed by Samuel Slipp to describe the child (usually the daughter) who attempts to rescue and hold the parents' marriage together by unconsciously accepting the projective identification of one parent (usually from the father) of the good-mother image. The spouse rejects this projection since it is not based on reality factors. This is most commonly seen in hysteric and borderline patients, where the daughter plays a nurturant mother-wife role to a narcissistic father (see parentification).

Guerin, Philip J., Jr.

American psychiatrist who was a student of Murray Bowen and an advocate of Bowenian family therapy. He has contributed to the history of family therapy in the chapter of his book, *Family Therapy: Theory and Practice*, Gardner, New York, 1976. He has had a long-term working relationship with Thomas Fogarty at the Center for Family Living in New Rochelle, New York.

Gurman, Alan S.

American psychologist and family researcher at the Department of Psychiatry, University of Wisconsin, where he is Director of the Psychiatric Outpatient Clinic and Coordinator of the Couples-Family Clinic. He published the first comprehensive review of marital therapy outcome research. He has published numerous papers and edited a number of books on family therapy: *Couples in Conflict*, with David Rice, Jason Aronson, New York, 1975; *Effective Psychotherapy: A Handbook of Research*, with David Kniskern, Pergamon, New York, 1977; *Questions and Answers in the Practice of Family Therapy*, Brunner/Mazel, New York, 1981; and *Handbook of Family Therapy*, with David Kniskern, Brunner/Mazel, New York, 1981.

Haley, Jay

American communications expert who was introduced into the Palo Alto Group by Gregory Bateson. Haley was strongly influenced by the work of the hypnotherapist, Milton H. Erickson. Haley developed from this the paradoxical approach in family therapy, with its focus on behavior change in short-term treatment. He also contributed to the double-bind theory along with Bateson, Jackson, and Weakland. In 1967, he joined Minuchin at the Philadelphia Child Guidance Clinic. He was the first editor of *Family Process* until 1969 and is the author of many papers and the books: *Strategies of Psychotherapy*, Grune and Stratton, New York, 1963; *Advanced Techniques of Hypnosis and Therapy: Selected Papers of Milton H. Erickson*, Grune and Stratton, New York, 1967; *Changing Families*, Grune and Stratton, New York, 1971; *Uncommon Therapy*, W. W. Norton, New York, 1973; *Problem-Solving Therapy*, Jossey-Bass, San Francisco, 1973; *Leaving Home*, McGraw-Hill, New York, 1980; and with L. Hoffman, *Techniques of Family Therapy*, Basic Books, New York, 1967.

hard-core family

A family beset with multiple problems with which it cannot cope and which usually are associated with socioeconomic deprivation. The family organization is disrupted and family members suffer unemployment, child neglect and abandonment, alcoholism, drug addiction, crime, and physical abuse. They are frequently involved with many social agencies around repeated crises.

Hoffman, Lynn

American psychologist who since the mid 1960s has worked closely with Jay Haley to develop strategic approaches in family therapy. She has written *Techniques of Family Therapy*, Basic Books, New York, 1967, with Jay Haley, comparing techniques of five different approaches to family therapy, and *Foundations of Family Therapy*, Basic Books, New York, 1981. She left the Philadelphia Child Guidance Clinic in 1975 to come to New York where she continued at the Downstate Medical Center and the Ackerman Institute for Family Therapy.

Howells, John G.

English psychiatrist who has pioneered the use of family psychiatry, taking the family as the unit of treatment, in hospital and outpatient services for all cases. He devised vector therapy in his work with families. He is Director of the Institute of Family Psychiatry at the Ipswich and East Suffolk Hospital, Ipswich,

England, and is the author of many articles and books in child psychiatry. He has also written *Theory and Practice of Family Psychiatry*, Brunner/Mazel, New York, 1971, and *Principles of Family Psychiatry*, Brunner/Mazel, New York, 1975.

identified patient

The family member who overtly manifests symptoms which are considered to stem from a larger network of dysfunctional family relationships. It is assumed that the symptomatic patient preserves family homeostasis and preserves the existing family system.

infantilization

A process wherein one or both parents interfere with the individuation and separation of a child, keeping the child dependent and immature.

integrative family therapy

A form of family therapy developed by Bunny S. Duhl and Frederick J. Duhl which examines at one time all the levels of the family system that determine behavior and attitudes to integrate individual developmental levels, family processes expectable and available in the member (taking into account the family life cycle), as well as the transactions and system patterns the family demonstrates.

interactional approach of the Mental Research Institute

Family interaction theory and practice of the Mental Research Institute had its foundation in the theories of Harry Stack Sullivan, Franz Alexander, Ludwig von Bertalanffy, as well as a number of philosophers (Russell, Whitehead, Wittgenstein, etc.). The goal is to change transactions and communication patterns in the dysfunctional family which affect the identified patient. Attention is paid to verbal and nonverbal behavior, its timing, and also the congruence between these two levels. The focus is on modification and change of behavior and not on cognitive insight or emotional catharsis. For example, the patient may be asked not to change (a paradoxical instruction) or pressured to change by making it contingent on continuation of therapy.

Jackson, Don D. (1920-1968)

American psychiatrist and psychoanalyst who was one of the founders of the Mental Research Institute in Palo Alto, California, also known as the Palo Alto Group. Jackson was trained psychoanalytically and was influenced by the work of Harry Stack Sullivan. He had completed his residency at Chestnut Lodge during the time Frieda Fromm-Reichman was there, and was then invited to join the Palo Alto Group by Gregory Bateson as the psychiatric consultant to their work with schizophrenic families. Jackson, along with Weakland, was the first to publish on the systematic use of conjoint family therapy with schizophrenic patients in an outpatient setting. His major contribution is the theory of family homeostasis, i.e., the induction of the identified patient to be the symptom bearer for the family in order to sustain the family's balance of relationship. He was also a major contributor to the double-bind theory of schizophrenia. His untimely death at a young age, just as his achievements were being rewarded, was a tragic loss to the field of family therapy.

joining

A term used in structural family therapy in which the therapist fits in with the family's organization and style. Unless the therapist can first join the family and use himself to be accepted and to establish a therapeutic alliance, the family organization cannot be explored to allow for later restructuring.

Journal of Marital and Family Therapy

The official organ of the American Association for Marriage and Family Therapy (AAMFT), which began publication in 1975. It was originally called the *Journal of Marriage and Family Counseling* and renamed in 1979 to its current title. The Journal's first editor was William C. Nichols, the editor until 1981 was Florence

Kaslow, and the current editor is Alan S. Gurman. Its Editorial Advisory Board contains many of the leaders in both fields of marital and family therapy. The Journal publishes articles on clinical practice, research, and theory.

Kadis, Asya (1901-1971)

American psychoanalyst prominent in the development of couples group therapy with Max Markowitz at the Postgraduate Center for Mental Health, New York. They considered couples groups, run by both a female and male co-therapist, as eliciting a greater number of parental and peer transferences, thus providing more opportunity to work these through.

Kaslow, Florence

American psychologist who has written extensively on divorce and divorce therapy and is the author of the book, *Supervision, Consultation, and Staff Training in the Helping Professions*, Jossey-Bass, San Francisco, 1977.

Kramer, Charles

American psychiatrist and psychoanalyst who organized and is Director, Center for Family Studies and the Family Institute of Chicago, which is one of the largest and most prestigious training centers for family therapy in the midwestern United States.

Laing, Ronald D.

English psychiatrist and psychoanalyst who was an early contributor and writer in the field of family therapy. He was influenced by existential and Marxist thinking in the development of his concept of mystification of the schizophrenic by his or her parents. This is defined as a misrepresentation of what is going on (process) or what is being done (praxis), which results in representing exploitation as a form of benevolence. Laing considered this as the preferred means by the parents of controlling the experience and action of the schizophrenic patient. His studies were done at the Schizophrenia and Family Research Unit of the Tavistock Institute of Human Relations, Langham Clinic, London. He is the author of *The Divided Self*, Tavistock, London, 1960; *The Self and Other*, Tavistock, London, 1961; with R. D. Cooper, *Reason and Violence: A Decade of Sartre's Philosophy—1950-1960*, Tavistock, London, 1964; and *Sanity, Madness, and the Family*, Tavistock, London, 1964.

Langsley, Donald G.

American psychiatrist and psychoanalyst who conducted at the Colorado Psychiatric Hospital one of the earliest, well designed studies of family therapy outcome research. This indicated that experimental groups, where patients and families received outpatient family crisis intervention, had superior results to the comparison groups, where the patient was hospitalized and received conventional individual treatment. Collaborators in this research were F. S. Pittman and P. Machotka. Langsley was Chairman of the Department of Psychiatry, University of Cincinnati, School of Medicine, Ohio, and President, American Psychiatric Association, 1980-1981.

La Perrière, Kitty

American psychologist who has been influenced by the work of Margaret Mahler and contributed to understanding parent-child relations in family therapy. She was, until 1980, Director of Education, Ackerman Institute for Family Therapy, New York City.

Laqueur, Peter (1909-1979) (See Group Therapy Section)

American psychiatrist who pioneered the development of multiple family therapy, which combined family and group therapy advantages. This was mostly used with hospitalized and post-hospitalized schizophrenic patients and their families.

ledger of merits (See contextual family therapy)

A term devised by Boszormenyi-Nagy which describes the ethical balance of parent-child relationships. The positive factors (resulting from mature, loving object relations, where the needs of the child are gratified) are balanced against the negative factors (where the child is manipulated and exploited for the narcissistic needs of the parents). The justice or relational integrity of human relations is examined in contextual family therapy.

Lewis, Jerry M.

American psychiatrist and family researcher who has studied functional and dysfunctional families (mid-range and severe) using multidimensional instruments at the Timberlawn Research Foundation in Texas. Differences in the types of disorders were correlated with power structure, degree of differentiation, communication, relationship (oppositional or affiliative), reality sense, affect, as well as attitude to change or loss. Mid-range families tended to be depressive, and severely dysfunctional families had a schizophrenic member. Results of the study are reported in the book co-authored with W. R. Beavers, J. T. Gossett, and V. A. Phillips, *No Single Thread: Psychological Health in Family Systems*, Brunner/Mazel, New York, 1976.

Lidz, Theodore

American psychiatrist and psychoanalyst who was one of the early founders of family therapy. His study of schizophrenic patients and their families contributed significantly to the theoretical understanding of this area. Starting at Johns Hopkins, he went to Yale in 1951 where he collaborated with Stephen Fleck and Alice R. Cornelison to publish widely, including the book, *Schizophrenia and the Family*, International Universities Press, New York, 1965. In schizophrenic families, it was noted there was disruption of generational boundaries, confusion of role relationships, and inadequate acculturation, i.e., poor development of language and coping skills for the patient to adapt outside the family. In some families, usually with women patients, the father was narcissistic, dominant, and demeaning toward the wife, forming an alliance with the daughter. Lidz labeled this family constellation "schism." In other families, the dominant parent (usually the mother) formed an alliance with the sick spouse (folie à famille), usually most damaging to male children. Lidz termed this "skew." Lidz has remained within the psychoanalytic movement and has published widely on the relationship of family studies to psychoanalytic theory.

loyalty system
A term devised by Ivan Boszormenyi-Nagy to describe a powerful force operating upon the behavior of individuals in a family. Each loyalty system can be characterized as an uninterrupted bookkeeping through the generations of obligations, with alternating positive and negative balances. For example, showing of concern and caring add to the positive balance, and any form of exploitation depletes it.

MacGregor, Robert
American psychiatrist who developed multiple impact therapy, initially with families having a delinquent adolescent. Families came to Galveston, Texas, for two days and were seen intensively in various combinations of its members and in various treatment modes—family, group, and individual. The family was then assigned tasks and role clarity was defined.

Madanes, Cloe
Codirector of the Family Therapy Institute established in Maryland in 1976 with her husband Jay Haley. She is the author of *Strategic Family Therapy*, Jossey-Bass, San Francisco, 1981.

marital contract
A term used by Clifford Sager to refer to each spouse's expressed and unexpressed, conscious and unconscious, concepts of his or her obligations within the marital relationship and the benefits he/she expects to derive in exchange. In therapy an explicit contract is worked out.

marital counseling
The therapeutic intervention whereby a trained counselor

works with married couples to resolve immediate problems and conflicts in their relationship. The spouses are seen together by the same counselor.

marriage
A socially sanctioned relationship between two adults. Marriage determines specific roles, involving reciprocal obligations, duties, as well as rights.

marriage (marital) therapy
A form of psychotherapy conducted by a therapist with the marital pair, aimed at improving the marital relationship, and attempting to alter the couple's psychodynamics and relationship. It is assumed marital partners select and/or shape their spouses to perpetuate their individual neurotic patterns which find expression interpersonally in marital conflict; the marital relationship also helps perpetuate individual pathology.

Martin, Peter A.
American psychiatrist who has been a pioneer in marital therapy. He is Clinical Professor of Psychiatry, University of Michigan, has published widely, and is the author of the book, *A Marital Therapy Manual*, Brunner/Mazel, New York, 1976.

McMaster Model of Family Functioning
A method of evaluating the effectiveness of family functioning that was developed by Nathan Epstein and his colleagues which includes problem-solving, communication, roles, affective responsiveness, affective involvement, and behavior control. It has been used extensively in research and in problem-solving systems family therapy.

Mental Research Institute (M.R.I.)
A group of family therapists and researchers in the western United States (Palo Alto, California) who shared responsibility for the development of family therapy. M.R.I. members have included Gregory Bateson, Don D. Jackson, Jay Haley, Virginia

Satir, and Paul Watzlawick. They are best known for the concepts of the double bind, family homeostasis, and brief family therapy.

metacommunication
A term devised by Gregory Bateson to denote a message about a message. It frames the content of the communication by conveying the sender's attitude toward the message, toward himself, and toward the receiver. Metacommunication can be nonverbal or verbal and can determine how a message will be received (see double bind).

metafamily
As defined by Clifford Sager, includes the remarried family and former spouses, grandparents, stepgrandparents, aunts, uncles, and others with significant input into the remarried system. Also called the REM suprasystem.

Midelfort, Christian F.
American psychiatrist who was one of the pioneers in the family therapy movement. In 1957 he published the book, *The Family in Psychotherapy*, McGraw-Hill, New York, and delivered the first psychiatric paper on family therapy technique at the 1952 meeting of the American Psychiatric Association.

Milan group
The Milan (Italy) Center for Family Studies has contributed to strategic family therapy especially in the areas of anorexia nervosa, encopresis, and schizophrenia. Organized by Mara Selvini Palazzoli, its principal members are Luigi Boscolo, Gianfranco Cecchin, and Guilana Prata.

Minuchin, Salvador
American psychiatrist and psychoanalyst who was trained in Argentina and in the early 1960s worked at the Wiltwyck School for Boys in New York. He became interested in the families of these delinquent boys and wrote the book with co-authors, B.

Montalvo, B. G. Guerney, B. L. Rosman and F. Schumer, *Families of the Slums*, Basic Books, New York, 1967. He became Director of the Philadelphia Child Guidance Clinic in 1967, inviting Braulio Montalvo from New York and Jay Haley from California to join him. An extensive training program was created and their unique form of treatment, structural family therapy, developed. The approach focuses on the here and now with the therapist playing an active, directive role, monitoring communication, and changing power structure and alliances. This approach has become one of the most influential forms of family therapy practiced in the United States. Minuchin and his colleagues have also contributed to the research and treatment of anorexia nervosa. Minuchin retired from the directorship of the Philadelphia Child Guidance Clinic in 1980.

His publications are numerous, including the books, *Families and Family Therapy*, Harvard University Press, Cambridge, 1974; *Psychosomatic Families: Anorexia Nervosa in Context* (with B. L. Rosman and L. Baker), Harvard University Press, Cambridge, 1978; and *Family Therapy Techniques* (with H. Charles Fishman), Harvard University Press, Cambridge, 1981.

Mishler, Elliot, G.

American psychologist who was one of the early researchers of family processes in normals and schizophrenia. Along with his collaborator, Nancy Waxler, he experimentally investigated the findings of Lidz, Wynne, and Bateson at Massachusetts Mental Health Center of Harvard Medical School in Boston. They have published the books, *Family Processes and Schizophrenia*, Science House, New York, 1968; and *Interaction in Families*, Wiley, New York, 1968.

Mittlemann, Bela (1899-1959)

American psychiatrist and psychoanalyst who was the first to publish a paper on the concurrent analyses of 12 marital partners, as well as stressing the importance of treating the spouse because of the complementary nature of the neurosis.

modeling

Family members identify with and imitate the adaptive behavior demonstrated by the therapist. If this behavior is rewarded by positive outcomes and repeated often enough, it may become incorporated into the patient's behavioral repertoire and be curative.

morphogenesis

A term from general systems theory to describe the processes in any system, including family systems, wherein deviation-amplifying tendencies to change are generated through positive feedback. It is characteristic of healthy families who are more spontaneous and less rigid than disturbed families, having a flexible structure, openness to growth, and responsiveness to new circumstances.

morphostasis

A term derived from general systems theory. Morphostasis refers to a deviation-correcting process (negative feedback) by which an individual's or system's behavior is brought back toward the "steady state" or equilibrium of the system. Homeostasis is a synonym by analogy from physiology.

Mosher, Loren

American psychiatrist and family researcher who is Director of the Center for Study of Schizophrenia, National Institute of Mental Health. He has been active in establishing, studying, and reporting on Soteria House, an alternative residential treatment center for acute schizophrenic patients. He has published very widely and is the editor with J. Gunderson of *Psychotherapy of Schizophrenia*, Jason Aronson, New York, 1975.

multigenerational transmission process

A concept of Murray Bowen in family therapy which defines the principle of projection of varying degrees of immaturity to different children in the family. The maximally involved child emerges with a lower level of self-differentiation. Three generations of this process are considered necessary for schizophrenia to evolve in a child.

multiple family (group) therapy (MFT or MFGT)

A form of therapy pioneered by Peter Laqueur in which three or more families usually gather together as a group with one or more therapists to discuss common problems. This form of treatment is considered to combine many of the assets of family as well as group therapy, especially universalizing a problem and offering group support.

multiple-impact therapy (MIT)

An intensive, brief (two or three days) form of therapy originated by Robert MacGregor with families who have an adolescent son or daughter in crisis and are unable to participate in conventional treatment programs because of time, distance, and/or economic factors. It starts with a team-family conference and includes multiple therapist situations, individual interviews, and group therapy, interspersed with brief staff conferences. Tasks are assigned and roles clarified.

multiple therapy

A form of combined treatment used by Carl Whitaker and Thomas Malone as well as others where a single patient is seen by two psychotherapists who make up a therapeutic unit. Interviews with the patient's family, including the patient, are also done jointly by both these therapists.

mutuality

A term introduced into family studies by Lyman Wynne to describe healthy relationships in which there is an awareness of each other's divergent needs and wishes and a willingness to accommodate to one another without loss of individuality, constriction, or fear.

mystification
A term devised by R. D. Laing to describe the confusion resulting in the schizophrenic due to misrepresentation of what is going on (process) or what is being done (praxis) by the parents, so that exploitation is presented as benevolence.

network family therapy (also called social network therapy [See Group Therapy Section])
A type of family therapy originated by Ross Speck that involves family members, the extended family, and also friends. It has been useful in diluting symbiotic binding of family members and providing an external social support network to mobilize resources.

nuclear family
Consists of a married man and woman with their child or children.

Oberndorf, Carl P. (1882-1954)
American psychiatrist and psychoanalyst who was first to report on folie à deux in a marriage, which pointed out the interaction of each spouse's neurosis to the other. He gave the first psychiatric report on marital therapy at the 1931 meeting of the American Psychiatric Association and in 1938 published on the consecutive individual psychoanalyses of five married couples.

oppositional symbiotic survival pattern
A term devised by Samuel Slipp to describe the negativistic relationship by which the child who becomes depressive achieves a measure of autonomy by passive-aggressively frustrating the pressure for achievement of a dominant parent. The dominant parent does not reward achievement, but rather exploits it for his or her own self-esteem. The dominant parent becomes internalized in the superego of the depressive and this form of interaction is then acted out transferentially with others.

Palazzoli Selvini (See Selvini Palazzoli)

Palo Alto Group (See Mental Research Institute)

paradoxical prescription (therapeutic double bind)
A directive used in strategic family therapy, whereby the therapist makes a statement to the family which overtly strengthens or promotes the family homeostatic defenses and does not arouse resistance. Yet this prescription reveals the secondary gain of the patient's symptomatic behavior for the family, hence *covertly* change is expected. An example would be to tell a son to continue to fail since in this way he is helping his father to feel good about himself.

parentification (parental child)
Describes the allocation of parental power and responsibility to a child. Normally, this occurs in large families or where parents work and an older child is given authority over younger children. Abnormally, this occurs when a parent abdicates his or her position of authority or assigns an adult role to a child, thereby breaching generational boundaries.

Paul, Norman
American psychiatrist who was influential in pioneering family therapy and multiple family therapy. He is particularly known for stressing the significance of unresolved grief in the parents as an etiological factor in the development of schizophrenia in the child. The parents do not acknowledge or mourn the loss they have suffered, resulting in a dread of abandonment, rigidity of family structure, and interference with the child's individuation and separation. He is Clinical Associate Professor with the Department of Neurology, Boston University School of Medicine. In 1965 he received the Edward Strecker Award and in 1966 the Public Broadcasting System's Peabody Award for his work with families. He is the author of numerous papers and the book, with Betty Paul, *A Marital Puzzle*, W. W. Norton, New York, 1975.

Pearce, John K.
American psychiatrist who has published extensively on the topic of ethnicity and family therapy. He is on the faculty of the Cambridge Family Institute, Cambridge, Massachusetts, and the co-editor with Leonard J. Friedman of the book, *Family Therapy: Combining Psychodynamic and Family Systems Approaches*, Grune and Stratton, New York, 1980.

Philadelphia group
An important center for training and research in family therapy at the Eastern Pennsylvania Psychiatric Institute (E.P.P.I.) under Ivan Boszormenyi-Nagy. Other members who have also made creative contributions to the field are Ray Birdwhistell, James Framo, David Rubenstein, Albert Scheflen, Geraldine Spark, and Ross Speck.

Postgraduate Center for Mental Health
Important psychotherapy training center in New York City and the largest outpatient psychiatric clinic in the United States, responsible for pioneering approaches in analytic group psychotherapy, couples and marital therapy. Its Divorce Mediation Center, through Linda Silberman (Professor of Family Law at New York University), achieved a landmark decision from the Association of the Bar of the City of New York legitimizing a lawyer's participating with a mental health professional in a nonprofit organization. Postgraduate members making contributions have included Alexander Wolf, Manny Schwartz, Asya Kadis, Max Markowitz, Nina Fieldsteel, Henry Kellerman, Zanvil Liff, Marvin Aronson, and Samuel Slipp.

premarital counseling
A form of counseling whereby a therapist works with a couple prior to marriage to deepen their understanding of one another and of the marital relationship, so as to help them decide for themselves whether to marry and what kind of marital decisions they may need to face.

problem-centered systems family therapy

A form of family therapy developed by Nathan B. Epstein and his colleagues at the Department of Psychiatry at McGill and McMaster Universities in Canada. Focus of the therapy is on the problems presented by the family, as well as those identified in the assessment stage. The McMaster Model of Family Functioning, which evaluates problem-solving, communication, roles, affective responsiveness, affective involvement, and behavior control, is used during this phase, since it defines critical areas of structure and function. A therapeutic contract is cooperatively agreed upon and treatment involves clarifying and resolving these problems collaboratively.

pseudohostility

A term used by Lyman Wynne to describe relationships that are formally like those of pseudomutuality, but the surface or presenting level of experience is one of constant bickering, blaming, and hostility, rather than harmony. In both forms of relatedness, genuine individuation and differentiation do not take place, are feared, and are avoided by maintenance of fixed mythic beliefs. However, in pseudohostility intimacy is also dreaded, so collusive acceptance of bickering forestalls both feared intimacy and feared separation.

pseudomutuality

A term devised by Lyman Wynne to describe enduring relationships, especially in families in which a discrepancy arises between strong wishes for relatedness and actual behavior or transactions. The discrepancy is ignored in further support of the "sense" of relatedness. In pseudomutual family relationships, the family myths often stress the dire consequences resulting from separation and deviation from family rules. There is a relatively limited number of fixed, engulfing family roles. The "sense" of family relationships is sustained with an illusion or facade of mutuality, but at the expense of individual identity and role differentiation of the members. Pseudomutuality, like double-bind relationships, refers to two simultaneous levels of functioning that often are sustained for long periods without overt distress, until the discrepancy between rules or beliefs and actual behavior becomes dysfunctional for the family system and/or the family members. Sometimes extreme forms of such dysfunctional discrepancies are symptomatically labeled as an acute schizophrenic or psychotic episode. However, pseudo-mutuality is also found in other families and relationships.

psychoanalytic family therapy

Concern with the social and cultural aspects of personality development and functioning was introduced into psychoanalytic theory by Alfred Adler and Carl Jung and later by Franz Alexander, Erich Fromm, Karen Horney, Abram Kardiner, Clara Thompson, and Harry Stack Sullivan. Influenced by these culturalists and neo-Freudian thinkers, many early analysts started working therapeutically with both spouses. (Indeed, Freud himself did concurrent marital therapy, it is reported.) Nathan W. Ackerman, Don D. Jackson, Theodore Lidz, and Murray Bowen, who pioneered family therapy, came from psychoanalytic backgrounds, as well as many of the current leaders in the field.

The aim of psychoanalytic family therapy is to establish a collaborative working alliance to explore the relationship of individual and interpersonal factors in the current relationships, providing insight into genetic and unconscious factors from past conflicts and helping the members to function more freely and authentically in terms of emotions and thoughts. Change occurs internally by working through old conflicts that influence current relationships. In other forms of directive family therapy, change is imparted from outside by providing solutions to problems, teaching skills, manipulating the power and communication structure, or through paradoxical prescriptions. It is assumed that change resulting from growth developing within the persons will result in greater and more permanent personality strength and individuation.

In marital therapy, Henry Dicks and James Framo have made important contributions. Ivan Boszormenyi-Nagy and Murray Bowen, although developing their own forms of therapy, stress genetic factors in exploring transmission of patterns through the generations as well as projective mechanisms. Other psychoanalytic family therapists who have made contributions are Ian Alger, Nathan Epstein, Leonard J. Friedman, Martin Grotjahn, Henry Grunebaum, Charles Kramer, Clifford Sager, Fred Sander, Samuel Slipp, John Spiegel, Helm Stierlin, and Israel Zwerling.

Ravich, Robert A.

American psychiatrist and family researcher who has contributed to the understanding of marital interaction through the use of the train game. The game was adopted for marital couples from Morton Deutsch's Acme Bolt Truck Game, used in social psychology to measure cooperative-competitive behavior. Ravich has been a prominent teacher of family therapy at New York Hospital for many years. He is the co-author with Barbara Wyden of the book, *Predictable Pairing*, Peter H. Wyden, New York, 1974.

Reiss, David

American psychiatrist, psychoanalyst, and family researcher who experimentally investigated individual, cognitive, and family interaction of normal, delinquent, and schizophrenic families. He noted that schizophrenic patients problem-solved better alone than with their families, and that these families were so "consensus sensitive" that premature closure occurred with the lowest level of problem-solving. Normals tended to do better in their families than when alone, and these families problem-solved the best. Delinquent families tended to be distant and isolated from one another and their problem-solving ability was between the two former groups. The original work was done at Massachusetts Mental Health Center, then at the National Institute of Mental Health, and continued at George Washington University.

remarried (REM) family

A remarried (REM, blended, reconstituted, or step-) family is formed by the marriage or living together of two adults, one or both of whom was widowed or divorced, with their custodial or visiting children.

Rome group
The Italian Society for Family Therapy located in Rome, Italy, which is lead by Maurizio Andolfi and includes Paolo Menghi, Anna Nicolo, and Carmine Saccer, is known for its combination of strategic and structural approaches with severely dysfunctional families.

rubber fence
A term used by Lyman Wynne to describe the boundary problem of families, often with a schizophrenic member, in which the family behaves as if it could be a completely self-sufficient, closed system. Persons who do not follow family rules (myths) are experienced as psychologically excluded, even biologic family members, whereas others may be temporarily or enduringly incorporated into the family system (for example, unwary family therapists). Thus the specific location of the family boundary may shift as if made of rubber, always encircling, without clearly defined gates for acceptable entry and exit.

Russell's Theory of Logical Types
Bertrand Russell's theory that was used by Gregory Bateson to develop the double-bind theory of schizophrenia. Russell postulates there is discontinuity between a class and its members, each being at a different level of abstraction, different logical types. In communication, the nonverbal message may be used to define the context of the verbal message, for example, playfulness vs. seriousness. In the double-bind theory it is postulated that the schizophrenic has not learned to handle these different level messages or signals, for example, confusing literal with metaphoric, and thus is unable to interpret and judge the meaning of communication.

Sager, Clifford
American psychiatrist and psychoanalyst whose broad con-

tributions have ranged from historian of the family therapy movement, his concept of the marriage contract, and his work with reconstituted (or step-) families. He is Director of Family Psychiatry, Jewish Board of Family and Children's Services, New York, and Clinical Professor of Psychiatry, New York Hospital-Cornell Medical Center.

Satir, Virginia

American social worker who started one of the earliest training programs in family therapy in 1959 at the Mental Research Institute, Palo Alto, California. In 1962, she received a five-year grant from the National Institute of Mental Health, the first federal training grant awarded for family therapy. Her concerns about self-esteem and other individual dynamics stemmed from her psychoanalytic training in Chicago. One of the earliest primers on how to do family therapy was written by her, *Conjoint Family Therapy: A Guide to Theory and Technique*, Science and Behavior Books, Palo Alto, 1964. In the mid-1960s she gradually disengaged from the Mental Research Institute and became active in the human growth movement. She has been one of the most charismatic and stimulating teachers of family therapy, traveling widely throughout the world to popularize family therapy. She also wrote the book, *Peoplemaking*, Science and Behavior Books, Palo Alto, 1972.

savior

A term used by Samuel Slipp to describe the child who is assigned the role of enhancing the family's social prestige. Projective identification of the good self into the child occurs and the parent(s) live vicariously through the child's achievements. This is felt to be pathogenic of depressive disorders (see also oppositional symbiotic survival pattern).

scapegoat

A term used by Norman Bell and Nathan Ackerman to describe the family member seen as bad or sick. The scapegoat, when a child, serves to displace aggression away from conflict between the parents, thereby preserving the marital relationship. The scapegoat can also be the *spouse*, as noted in schizophrenic families by Theodore Lidz and in families with an hysteric or depressive by Samuel Slipp.

Scheflen, Albert E. (1920-1980)

American psychiatrist, psychoanalyst, and pioneering family researcher who came to the Eastern Pennsylvania Psychiatric Institute in 1960. With Ray Birdwhistell he studied through microanalysis of sound motion pictures the subtle linguistic, paralinguistic, kinesic (or facial-postural) behavioral forms of interaction during individual psychotherapy and later family therapy. The method used was termed "context analysis" which was ethnographic and descriptive and not involved in experimental methodology or isolating and counting single variables. Behavior was studied directly in its sequential relationship to the behavior of others. These subsystems are then integrated into larger transactions. Considerable control, monitoring, or regulation of interaction was found and the nonlexical forms of how this was communicated were noted. Some aspects that were studied were quasi-courtship responses (preening), disapproval responses (nosewiping), gaze-holding, parallelism (identical postures), syncrony of movement, etc., which regulated alliances, interpersonal distance, and communication.

Scheflen continued his research studies at Bronx State Hospital and was Professor of Psychiatry, Albert Einstein School of Medicine.

schism

A term devised by Theodore Lidz to describe one form of interaction in some families with a schizophrenic child (most often a daughter). The parents live in a chronic state of severe discord and fail to achieve complementarity of needs. Because of this, there is undercutting of the spouse's worth and a tendency to compete for and form alliances with the children, thereby breaching generational boundaries.

Selvini Palazzoli, Mara

Italian psychiatrist, founder of the Milan Center for Family Studies in Italy. Her work in strategic family therapy has resulted in helping develop this brief therapy approach into a significant movement in the field. Her published work has been primarily with anorexia, encopresis, and schizophrenia, resulting in many papers and the books, *Self-Starvation*, Jason Aronson, New York, 1978; and with L. Boscolo, G. Cecchin and G. Prata, *Paradox and Counterparadox*, Jason Aronson, New York, 1978.

sibling position

Alfred Adler was one of the first to describe how certain personality characteristics are often determined by birth order. Elaborating on this, Walter Toman describes ten personality profiles of sibling positions which can be used to assume the possible family process of past generations and in the present family. An example would be the overly responsible firstborn child who may assume parental functions. See Toman's *Family Constellation*, Springer, New York, 1961.

sibling subsystem

A term used in structural family therapy to describe the grouping of children within a family. Children learn peer relationships involving support, isolating, scapegoating, negotiating, cooperation, and competition. The boundaries of the sibling subsystem protect the children from adult intrusion.

Singer, Margaret

American psychologist and family researcher who worked with Lyman Wynne on communication patterns in families with a schizophrenic patient. In examining communication patterns of families, they have been able to predict the nature of the child's psychopathology. The "attention scale" devised by Singer and Wynne was found particularly valuable by other investigators who studied family therapy process. In recent years she has studied brainwashing procedures by cults.

skew

A term devised by Theodore Lidz to describe another form of interaction in some families with a schizophrenic child. The serious psychopathology of one marital partner is supported by the spouse, resulting in the distorted ideation being accepted in the family (folie à famille). There is considerable masking of conflict, creating an unreal atmosphere that does not help the child to trust his or her perception and judgment or learn social adaptive skills.

skill-training program for couples and families

A form of educational training or enrichment for couples and families, alone or in groups, which facilitates functioning but does not attempt to therapeutically change structure. Examples of existing programs are parent effectiveness training or teaching couples how to fight nondestructively. A skill-training program involves issues facing couples before marriage, during marriage (such as marriage encounters), parenting, the family, and divorce. Luciano L'Abate has written on this area extensively.

Skynner, A. C. Robin

English psychiatrist who was influenced by the group analyst, S. H. Foulkes, during training at the Maudsley Hospital, to apply group methods to working with children and their parents. His work has also been shaped by neo-Freudian psychoanalytic and object relations theories. He began the Institute of Family Therapy in London and is its Chairman. He is also a member of the Group-Analytic Practice. Skynner has had a deep interest in family process research and included these findings in his theory and work with families. He is the author of many papers and the book, *Systems of Family and Marital Psychotherapy*, Brunner/Mazel, New York, 1976.

Slipp, Samuel

American psychiatrist and psychoanalyst who trained in family therapy in 1962 at the Mental Research Institute and was influenced by Don D. Jackson and Virginia Satir. He introduced object relations theory into family therapy using the primitive defense of projective identification, splitting, and idealization as a bridge between individual and interpersonal dynamics. His major concepts are the symbiotic survival pattern of family interaction in schizophrenia and the double bind over achievement in depression.

He has also contributed to the research literature on outcome studies of family therapy with Kenneth Kressel, and published experimental tachistoscopic studies with S. Nissenfeld, exploring his own family theory and other psychoanalytic theories of depression. He had been Director, Group and Family Therapy, New York University—Bellevue Medical Center since 1968, and since 1979 has been Medical Director, Postgraduate Center for Mental Health.

Sluzki, Carlos E.

American psychiatrist and psychoanalyst who was born in Argentina. He was a research associate of the Mental Research Institute in Palo Alto since 1965 and is its current Director. He has published extensively and serves on five editorial boards of journals and on the Board of Directors of the American Family Therapy Association. He is editor of the journal, *Family Process*.

Soteria House

An alternative community residential treatment center located in San Jose, California for schizophrenic patients which is operated by the Mental Research Institute, the Family Research and Training Center, and funded by the National Institute of Mental Health (N.I.M.H.). Loren Mosher of the N.I.M.H. Center for the Study of Schizophrenia was the consultant. A matched sample of schizophrenic patients was compared to residential drug treatment at the county hospitals.

Speck, Ross V.

American psychiatrist who has worked at the Eastern Pennsylvania Psychiatric Institute and developed the short-term family-network therapy. In order to diminish overdependency in the family and mobilize outside resources, the extended family, friends, neighbors, and others involved with the family are invited to the family's home. They meet together as a whole and in subgroups to provide a social support system. He is the author of many papers on technique in family therapy, as well as the author with C. Attneave of the book, *Family Networks*, Vintage, New York, 1973.

Spiegel, John P.

American psychiatrist, psychoanalyst, and family researcher who was strongly influenced by Florence Kluckholn's cultural anthropology and whose concepts about cultural-value orientations were utilized in studying various ethnic families. Spiegel also studied forms of conflict resolution in the family and role structure. He organized the first panel on family research in March 1957 at the American Orthopsychiatric Association meeting. His application of general systems theory to studying the relation of various levels of psychopathology and family functioning was presented in his book, *Transactions*, Science House, New York, 1971. Spiegel has been Director, Lemberg Center for the Study of Violence, Brandeis University, since 1966. He was President, American Psychiatric Association, 1979-1980, appointed Vice President, American Family Therapy Association at its inception, and is currently President, American Academy of Psychoanalysis.

stepfamily

Formed by the marriage or living together of two adults, one or both of whom was widowed or divorced, with their custodial or visiting children.

Stierlin, Helm

German psychiatrist and psychoanalyst who worked with Lyman Wynne at the National Institute of Mental Health and collaborated with Ivan Boszormenyi-Nagy. His early work involved studying the family interaction in schizophrenia including symbiotic relationships and binding of the patient's ego, superego, or id out of fear of annihilation or disloyalty to parental delegation. In a family, one child may be selected and delegated to fulfill a certain function for a parent. Stierlin is the author of a large number of papers and the books, *Conflict and Reconciliation*, Science House, New York, 1969; *Separating Parents and Adolescents*, Quadrangle, New York, 1974; *Adolph Hitler: A Family Perspective*, Psychohistory Press, New York, 1977; *Psychoanalysis and Family Therapy*, Jason Aronson, New York, 1977, and *The First Interview with the Family*, Brunner/Mazel, New York, 1980. He is Director of Family Therapy at the University of Heidelberg and editor of the journal, *Familiendynamik*.

strategic family therapy

A brief form of family therapy devised by Jay Haley and Richard Rabkin. Recent extensions in this form of therapy have been made by Mara Selvini Palazzoli and colleagues in Milan, Italy, where a family is interviewed by one or two therapists and also may be observed through a one-way mirror by one or more therapists. After deliberation by the therapist(s) (and observers), the family may be given a directive or a "paradoxical prescription" which overtly goes along with the pathology, does not disrupt family homeostasis, and enlists the family's own need for change. Sometimes the family's oppositionalism may be harnessed in the service of change. This approach has been used in anorexia nervosa, neurotic and psychotic disorders.

structural family therapy

A form of therapy developed by Salvador Minuchin focusing on changing the communication, functioning, and power structures of the family so as to alter symptomatic behavior in the identified patient. A change in family interaction is considered to bring about changes in individual behavior of family members. The focus is ahistoric, in the here and now, with the therapist playing an active role, monitoring communication, even rearranging seating to change structure and functioning of the family.

subsystems in the family

The family system as a whole is differentiated into a variety of smaller units that serve certain functions—dyads such as husband-wife, mother-father, mother-child, or child-child. Subsystems are also formed by generation, by sex, by interest, or by function. Individuals belong to a number of subsystems, but in each subsystem different levels of power exist for that person.

symbiotic survival pattern

A term devised by Samuel Slipp to describe a form of family interaction in which each member feels his self-esteem and survival is dependent on the behavior of the other. Each member thus feels omnipotent over, as well as helpless and controlled by, the other. This family pattern reinforces fixation at the symbiotic phase of development, prevents object constancy, individuation, and separating, as well as interfering with resolution of primary process thinking. In schizophrenia, the symbiotic binding mostly involves the ego and controls feelings, thoughts, and actions. In depression, the symbiotic binding involves the superego, with pressure for and against achievement. In hysteria, the symbiotic binding involves the id with eroticization of relationships.

symbolic-experiential family therapy

A form of family therapy developed by Carl A. Whitaker which considers change as coming primarily from experiential learning and self-evaluation. Insight into genetic factors is not considered necessary to change; however, interactional insights related to the here and now of treatment are valued. Co-therapy is encouraged, since it also provides a model or "meta-experience" for the family. Interpretations are most valuable when they are metaphorical and symbolically made about family relationships—using humor, teasing, fantasy, or free association to challenge the family's method of resolving stressful situations

Whitaker has used "acting crazy" as a therapeutic tool, utilizing irrelevant phrases or free associative fantasy during the session. This is seen to work in the same way as regression in the service of the ego, i.e., controllable and reversible. In the process, the family is forced to assume the "sane" component, in addition to the therapist serving as an example, giving the patient or the family permission to remain crazy under controlled circumstances. Whitaker also stresses the importance of the therapist being inconsistent—being a change agent. This undermines the rigid style of functioning of the family and prevents the therapist from following a technique mechanically.

symmetrical family interaction

An interaction with the family in which behaviors exhibited are similar. For example, anger is exchanged for anger. (See opposite term: complementary family interaction.)

systems theory

Systems theory refers to both general systems theory, a general scientific theory developed by Von Bertalanffy (see general systems theory), as well as to the family therapy approach formulated by Murray Bowen (see family systems theory). General systems theory was introduced into family therapy by the Palo Alto Group (Bateson, Jackson, etc.) as a way of relating the interaction of the family and the individual, as well as seeing how the homeostasis of the family system is maintained through negative feedback loops (morphostasis).

therapeutic contract in family therapy

The family and therapist, at the start of therapy, come to an agreement on the nature of the problem and on the goals for treatment. This contract may or may not have a clearly defined objective, but it must be initially agreed upon, even though at a future time it can be changed.

trading of dissociations

A term devised by Lyman Wynne to describe an interlocking network of perceptions about others based on dissociations about oneself in which each person projects the totality of a particular quality or feeling onto another family member, and in exchange allows the other to project unacceptable qualities onto himself or herself.

triangle (triad)

A three-person system described by Murray Bowen as the smallest stable relationship in the family. In periods of calm, the triangle is made up of an uncomfortable distant outsider and two close individuals. The outsider strives for closeness with one of the others. In periods of stress, the outside position is the most comfortable and most desired position. There are varying triangular patterns in the family that overlap one another. One of the most basic or common patterns results from tension between parents, with the father gaining the outside position and distancing from the mother. The child then becomes triangulated into a close alliance with the mother.

undifferentiated family ego mass

A term devised by Murray Bowen referring to the family's lack of separateness, consisting of a fused cluster of egos of individual family members as if they all had a common ego boundary. The ego fusion is the most intense in the least mature families, but fusion is present to some degree in all families. (See also enmeshment; symbiotic survival pattern.)

vector therapy

A form of family therapy described by John Howells whose aim is to modify adverse, negative emotional influences playing on individual family members, and to make these forces positive and nurturing.

Watzlawick, Paul

American psychologist and psychoanalyst born in Austria; one of the early members of the Mental Research Institute who was trained in Jungian analysis. He published many papers on communication, change, brief therapy, etc., and with J. H. Beavin and Don D. Jackson authored the book, *Pragmatics of Human Communication*, W. W. Norton, New York, 1967; with J.

Weakland and R. Fisch, *Change*, W. W. Norton, New York, 1974; *How Real is Real*, Random House, New York, 1976; with J. Weakland, *The Interactional View: Studies at the Mental Research Institute 1965-74*, W. W. Norton, New York, 1977; and *The Language of Change: Elements of Therapeutic Communication*, Basic Books, New York, 1978.

Whitaker, Carl A. (See symbolic-experiential family therapy)

American psychiatrist, one of the early founders of family therapy who, working with John Warkentin in 1943, started introducing members of the family into the treatment session besides the patient. In 1958, he published one of the first papers on conjoint marital therapy. He organized the first meeting of family therapists in 1953 inviting Gregory Bateson, Don Jackson, John Rosen and Albert Scheflen to Atlanta, Georgia. His theoretic orientation was influenced by Melanie Klein, Fred Allen, and Jung, as well as cultural anthropology. His early work was also with schizophrenics and their families. Minimizing the importance of insight, he used nonverbal and experiential techniques, at times acting whimsically, inconsistently, or crazily in the service of the therapeutic process. He has continued his work at the University of Wisconsin.

Wynne, Lyman C.

American psychiatrist and social psychologist, one of the pioneers of family therapy who made important theoretical contributions to the study of schizophrenic patients and their families. Having obtained a Ph.D. in the Department of Social Relations at Harvard (after his M.D.), he was influenced by the work of Talcott Parsons. Going to the National Institute of Mental Health in 1952, he studied schizophrenic patients and their families, noting that the role structure was too rigid, loose, or ambiguously defined. Relationships were too distant or too engulfing, lacking what Wynne termed a "cognitive focal distance." Communication was fragmented with shifts in content and attention. A facade of role complementarity existed, which he termed "pseudomutuality," or conflict to avoid intimacy, which he termed "pseudohostility." The family also prohibited relationships with the outside community, isolating its members in what Wynne termed a "rubber fence." He was on the first board of editors of the journal, *Family Process*. In 1971 he moved to the University of Rochester Medical School, where he became Chairman of the Department of Psychiatry.

Zuk, Gerald H.

American psychologist who developed go-between family therapy in which the therapist takes a mediating role in changing pathogenic, repetitive family patterns. In go-between therapy, the therapist identifies the problem, establishes a contract and then assumes the role of mediator (go-between). The therapist may at times take sides judiciously in order to change the existing homeostatic balance and the positions of family members.

Zwerling, Israel

American psychiatrist and psychoanalyst whose training analyst was Nathan W. Ackerman, with whom he later became a close friend. Zwerling began teaching family therapy at the Day Hospital Service of the Department of Psychiatry, Albert Einstein College of Medicine, which developed at Bronx State Hospital into one of the outstanding Family Studies Sections in the United States. Many leading teachers of family therapy developed from this Section including Chris Beels, Andrew Ferber, Thomas Fogarty, Philip Guerin, Harry and Marilyn Mendelsohn, and Fred Sanders. Albert Scheflen did a great deal of his research at Bronx State Hospital. Zwerling currently is Chairman, Department of Psychiatry, Temple University School of Medicine, Philadelphia.